LAUREN CANDIES TARPLEY

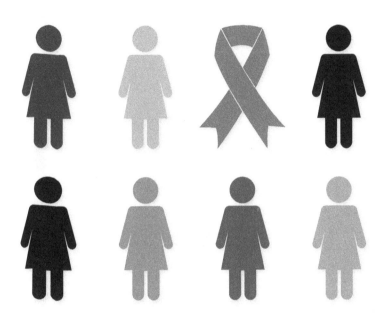

TYPE A
GUIDE
TO CANCER

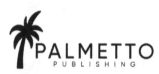

Charleston, SC
www.PalmettoPublishing.com

Type A Guide to Cancer

Copyright © 2021 by Lauren Tarpley

All rights reserved.

First Edition

Hardcover ISBN: 978-1-63837-634-7
Paperback ISBN: 978-1-63837-635-4
eBook ISBN: 978-1-63837-636-17

TYPE A
GUIDE
TO CANCER

Someone special thought you could use this book.

To: _____

From: _____

To: _____

From: _____

To: _____

From: _____

To: _____

From: _____

To: _____

From: _____

Dedications

To my dearest Trey, I want to thank you for always telling me that I can do anything I put my heart and mind to. You have always been my biggest cheerleader, and for that I will always be grateful and in awe of your love and endless support.

Chip, I want to thank you for allowing me to be your mother and thank you for showing me that I can do anything.

I want to thank my parents and sister for giving this little black girl one of the best childhoods, some of the best memories and support systems, still to this day, anyone could ask for. The way you raised us showed us that we can do whatever we put our minds to. I want to thank you for raising us to go after what we deserve and what our wildest dreams are made of.

Dr. Ebony Jade Hilton, thank you adopting me as your little sister and loving me unconditionally. You wrote the handbook on friendship and women supporting women. I am honored to call you family.

Jennifer and Claire, thank you for encouraging me to be my truest and most authentic self no matter what in the most important and formative years in my life.

Latha Bell, my angel, we are connected in yet another way now. I miss you every single day, and I am not sure what I would give to talk to you and hug you one more time, but when I am at my weakest, I think of you and the endless love that I still hold for you in my heart—and that gives me strength.

Carl and Debbie, thank you for treating me as your own daughter, from day one, and always supporting me.

To Emily and Kirby, I hate that you had this disease as well but thank you for being a beacon for me and answering all the questions I had and have about treatment and recovery.

This book is also dedicated to anyone who was ever told they could not do something. That includes a cancer diagnosis. They do not tell you that you cannot do it when you are diagnosed, but when you hear the words "It is cancer," you get that gut punch. Then after everything is laid out, the odds seem stacked against you. To that I say, "May the odds forever be in your favor."

You are not alone and are loved. You may not think that you need to hear that, but you do.

I promise to be real and honest with you through this book. It may not always be pretty, and it may get a little heavy, but it will usually circle back to a chuckle. These are my experiences and my journey, and some of it will be specific to breast cancer and being a black woman, but some of it will relate to being a cancer patient (in America) more generally.

Stay strong.
xxo
Lauren

Table of Contents

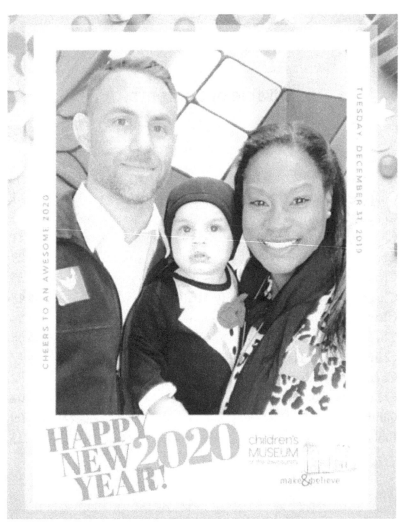

My family NYE 2019

CHAPTER 1:

Intro

Five…four…three…two…one…

Happy New Year! Twenty-twenty is going to be the *ish*! Twenty-nineteen was *so* good, 2020 can only be better!

Spoiler alert: 2020 was not the ish; it was just shit. There was a pandemic; my grandfather died (my last grandparent); I started a podcast—that last part was good. Oh, and I got cancer!

But let's back it up a bit. My name is Lauren, I am from Charleston, SC, and I am known for being heard before I am seen, at times. In my twenties (a.k.a. the "invincible years") I was a party girl and the life of the party. I worked by day and partied at night; if there was a barstool to be warmed, I was there. I was like Batman, but instead of a bat symbol they had a symbol of a martini glass that they would shine in the night sky, and I would appear! You know the motto "I'll sleep when I'm dead"? In those days, my body was literally held together by Sugar-Free Red Bull, hair extensions, tapas, purple eyeshadow, and vodka sodas.

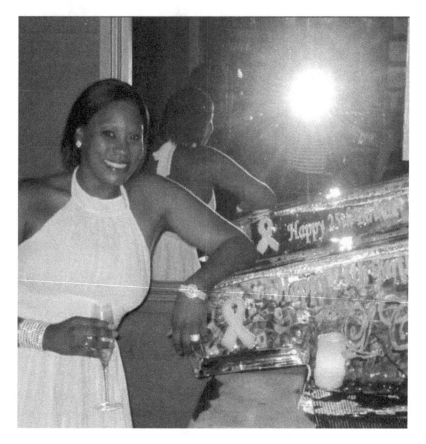

My 25th birthday party

I called my twenties the "invincible years" because I made mistakes, learned personal boundaries, and figured out who I was. I lived, loved, and learned a lot of things, and I traveled. I love traveling! Isn't that what your twenties are for?

I am slightly ashamed to admit that there was a short time where I did not have health insurance in my twenties, but it was a different time. We are talking about ten years ago. There was always the inherent sense of invulnerability; you go to work, you go out at night, you get a little sleep, and if you pop a multivitamin and occasionally eat an apple, you are supposed to be ok, right? I did not know about deductibles and out-of-pocket maximums. I did not know about HSAs, FSAs, or the like.

Toward the end of my twenties, I figured I should tighten things up and get other things together. I worked on my career, and I figured other things would fall into place, and they did. I met my husband at the age of twenty-eight, I got another job that offered health insurance, and I found a primary care provider. I was on top of the world. I felt great about the changes that I had made, and I felt even better that I had chosen to make them on my own timeline.

We got married, we had a son—the namesake we had always wanted—and I finally got a job at my (local) dream company, which I had been applying to work for off and on for about sixteen years. Things were going very well.

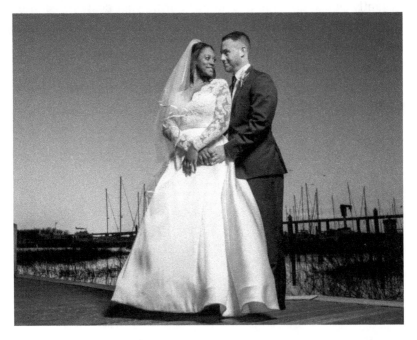

"Our Wedding Day" By Claire Hart

I started my new job at a new company in a new industry when my son was just four and a half months old. I had a slight battle with postpartum anxiety, but there was just a lot going on at the time. I will never forget the day I signed up for benefits at my new job. I had started, and it was extensive. I was hungry, so I put a pin in signing up and went downstairs for lunch. I had never worked at a company that had multiple floors. I often took the stairs for a little extra exercise. I was on the last half flight of stairs, and I blew out my flip-flop. I fell down the stairs! I was shocked, embarrassed, and instantly needed to make sure I had not seriously injured myself. Thank God no one was around. I hobbled to the café, got my lunch, and hoofed it back to my desk. While eating my lunch, I finished signing up for benefits. One of the insurance add-ons was a critical illness indemnity. The example they used was a broken leg and lost wages due to that. Having just had my life flash before my eyes and nearly broken my neck and leg, I instantly signed up. Think about that during your next open enrollment. You never know what lies around the corner. Just make sure it makes sense financially for you.

As time went by, things were just normal. Like you want. "No news is good news." But as the adage goes, "If you want to make God laugh, tell him your plans."

CHAPTER 2:

AYA

9.21.20

I am a daughter, sister, wife, mother, friend, baker, joke maker, hard worker, and sometimes an ass. When I thought of cancer and how it would directly affect me, for some reason I always thought I would get cancer, but I just always thought I would be old. I envisioned being in my late sixties or seventies and that we would be so technologically evolved as a society at that point that it would be a single doctor appointment or single surgery that would take care of it. I never lived in fear of cancer; I always thought of it in obscurity. I never thought that I would get cancer at the time I was looking to have a second baby or that I would be an AYA cancer patient.

Adolescent and young adult (AYA) cancer is any cancer that impacts a person aged fifteen to thirty-nine at the time of diagnosis. Care for AYA cancer is best when it is separated from both children and older adult cancer care, as AYA patients share unique medical and psychological challenges (UCLA Health 2021).

AYA cancer patients and survivors are the most underserved patient population by age and are also more likely to receive a late diagnosis or to be misdiagnosed, compared to other age groups. Patients, and even their doctors, often do not consider cancer because of how "rare" it is for this age group. Medical debt or even bankruptcy are realities for AYAs in the US (Stupid) Cancer 2021)

"About 89,000 young people [age fifteen to thirty-nine] are diagnosed with cancer each year in the United States—accounting for about five percent of cancer diagnoses in the United States. This is about eight times the number of cancers diagnosed in children ages 0 to 14 and about one twentieth, or five percent, of the number of cancers diagnosed in adults 40 years and older, based on Cancer Facts and Figures Exist Disclaimer 2020 by the American Cancer Society" (National Cancer Institute 2020).

"Certain cancers, such as primary bone cancer, Hodgkin lymphoma and testicular cancer, are most frequently diagnosed among adolescents and young adults. However, the incidence of specific cancer types varies according to age. Lymphomas and thyroid cancer are the most common cancers among 15- to 24-year-olds. Among 25- to 39-year-olds, breast cancer and thyroid cancer are the most common, based on NCI's Surveillance, Epidemiology, and End Results Program (SEER) Cancer Stat Facts" (National Cancer Institute 2020).

As an AYA cancer patient, I felt all these things—I felt unheard, I felt too young to be in this position, I felt sad, confused, and lost. No one else is going to fight for you the way you will fight for your own life; you must advocate for yourself. Thank God I have a fantastic primary care provider (PCP). He asked me the appropriate questions and determined that I was a candidate for diagnostic and preventative mammograms. But initially I felt slightly stupid asking my PCP for a referral for a mammogram at thirty. I felt interrogated when I went in for the procedures.

"How old are you?"

"Why are you here?"

"Does this run in your family?"

"Do you have a lump?"

"What is your birthday again?"

There is also the isolation. As an AYA cancer patient, you are not a pediatric cancer patient or an older cancer patient. Your friends are moving on with their lives, graduating high school and college. Getting married, having children, going on vacation or out to dinner. Meanwhile back at the ranch, you are in the chemo suite, having surgery or stuck at home because you are immunocompromised, and you do not want to get sick or risk having treatment pushed back. This is not the experience for everyone, but these are common IVF experiences among AYA cancer patients.

You are faced with your own mortality at a young age, whereas many never have to face that kind of trauma. That is a torturous experience that can stay with you for some time, if not forever. I know that my personal experience has been filled with anguish, stress, and confusion. I have lost "friends," and a year of my life along this journey, but at the same time, I have gained more than I lost.

When I thought of people who had abandoned their "friends" that have been diagnosed with cancer, at first, I just thought of them as terrible and selfish people. But as I thought it through a little more and analyzed it in my personal experience, I realized they simply just could not handle cancer. The people that I have lost or finally cut loose have never had anything bad happen to them. I say this with kindness and a tiny bit of jealousy. When I say nothing bad, I do not mean they have never had a breakup or a hangover; I mean they have never had a *life*-altering or *life*-ending event. For the people that could not handle *my* cancer—that is *their* problem. Their trauma response is flight. And I do not blame or even hate them for leaving, ghosting, or not even having the common courtesy to send a checkup text—although this lack of blame does not undo this harm. But again, I had to realize that that was not on me. That is on them. If my diagnosis scared them and they no longer wanted to be around me, I get it. It scared me too. But if you cannot holster that to be there for someone, you should grow up a little bit.

Being the eldest daughter of a woman who is the second youngest of seven, I have had many family members pass. I went to funerals as a child. Conversely, I know people my age that have not even lost a grandparent.

I look at old photos. Some pictures of me before diagnosis look like me and feel like me. Some look like me but look hollow. Like my soul is missing. Others do not look like me at all. I do and do not know who I am anymore. I like some things I used to and do not care for other things I did. Same with people. When I was diagnosed, I knew whom to reach out to, and I kind of had a feeling about people who would not be around after the hair fell out. In the last year, I have realized that it is not me or my growth that has scared people off. For the first time ever, it really is not me. It is their preconceived notions of cancer or their past experiences or traumas with cancer. Maybe they lost someone close to them to cancer, and they do not want to lose you. Maybe they do not want to hear the pain you are going through during treatment! Either way I have been left behind and ghosted by friends both old and new, and that was a lesson learned the hard way. It just reinforced my initial thought not to tell everyone about my diagnosis.

To further protect my heart (of glass, protected by stone), I decided to keep it a little close to the chest. Those actions of others made me feel dirty. I felt used up and like I was being discarded. That is where your support system comes in. If you get life-changing news and you lose your hair and go through treatment but nothing else changes (i.e., your friends and things), then it is easier. But I felt like Pig Pen from Peanuts. I felt like there was a weird film on me. I felt like others could see it or smell it and maybe that was why they did not want to be around me or want to support me through this. I felt marked for death. I felt like I had found something that was not supposed to be found that in turn saved my life. I do not know who I thought was eventually out for me, but I went through a period of time where I was just getting increasingly more scared of everything. The strong woman who had demanded the mammogram that got me in this situation had been scared into submission and herded away.

The first person on TV I recall seeing with cancer was Diem from *The Real World*. She would be weak at times, but from what I can remember, she went into remission, and then I saw her on the *Challenge*, and she was all over the place. All in all, I would say she was a great AYA cancer role model. She pushed through, and in my generation, and for me, she destigmatized AYA cancer.

I have struggled a lot with what and how much to share about my diagnosis, journey, and treatment. To be honest, in the beginning I was so scared to type one word about any of this. I did not want to speak a more aggressive situation into existence, but also, in the beginning it was very hard to even think about. Every thought ended in my dying, leaving my husband, son, and family without a Lauren.

I am in a better place now to be able to talk about it, but I have not really shared any of this on my personal social media. I am usually a liberal sharer (and at times an oversharer), but I just could not think or even talk about it without breaking down. I have found my voice and figured out how I would like to convey the message. This may be common in other cultures and races, but a lot of African Americans do not share a lot of their medical information, and rightfully so. There has been a longstanding mistrust between African Americans and the medical community (see the Tuskegee Study from 1932). But keeping my breast cancer diagnosis to myself after being diagnosed in my mid-thirties does not help anyone. I believe that one of the reasons for all of this is for me to help.

If the two women (Kirby and Emily) that I knew personally before my diagnosis had not been so open and forthright with their diagnosis and journey when they were also diagnosed as AYA cancer patients, I would not have had a support system or knew what on Earth to do or where to start. A lot of people in the AYA cancer age bracket do not really think about it, and sometimes you need to see someone who looks like you or you identify with to help you realize representation matters.

Journaling really helped but looking into statistics and learning *more* than what my doctors had told me did more damage than good. Also, personally for me, group therapy, especially virtually, due to the pandemic, did not work for me. If I do group therapy, I need for everyone in the group to be at my same stage and have my same mutation. I went to one group therapy session, and there were people in the group with different cancers and more aggressive cancers, and having been newly diagnosed, that just was not helpful for me. But since, I have found a personal oncological therapist, and that has made a world of difference.

CHAPTER 3:

Diagnosis

I have been getting mammograms since I was thirty. There is a moderate amount of cancer in my family, and I never wanted to be caught off guard and blindsided with a diagnosis. I thought that if I got mammograms on my own terms and when I thought necessary, I would not be caught off guard.

I was wrong.

I went in for my mammogram in July. I had a referral from January but due to how long it takes for a mammogram appointment, as well as the pandemic, I was not able to go any sooner.

I was thirty-four. I walked in—and if you know, you know that when you check in for a mammogram or a procedure at the hospital, then at every intersection, they ask you your name and birth date. The response was most commonly "Oh, girl, you are too young to be here. You do not need a mammogram for at least another six years. If you would like to leave, you can. We will not charge you." No one was ever rude; the only thing that I can come up with is that they just did not want me to waste anyone's time.

Up to this point I had had three mammograms. Everything was clear. I did receive letters post mammogram that I had dense breast tissue, but there were no areas of concern, and I was never called back.

This time was different. I was called the next day, and I was told that I had calcifications and asymmetry. Breast calcifications are calcium deposits within breast tissue. They appear as white spots or flecks on a mammogram. Breast calcifications are common on mammograms, and they are especially prevalent after age fifty. They were slightly concerned because I was sixteen years younger than the average patient with calcifications. They wanted me to come back for a second mammogram and an ultrasound this time. At the follow-up appointment, during the ultrasound the doctor did not like the look of the calcifications and ordered a biopsy. I had never had a biopsy before, but I called some friends, and they had, so I wasn't worried. It took a little time for the follow-up appointments and biopsies. I ended up getting the biopsy on September 3.

The doctor that day told me that the biopsy device would make a large click and would not hurt but in the following days it would feel like a punch in the face or the breast. I know a lot of people would be scared in this situation and just shrug that off or take it at face value, but I asked, "Have you ever been punched in the face?"

He said he had not.

So, I asked, "How do you know what being punched in the face feels like? Furthermore, have you ever had a biopsy in your large, dense breast?"

Again, he said, "No."

I was not surprised at his reaction. Not a ton of people who have been punched in the face or breast openly talk about it!

I did not give him too much crap, but these laughs and that conversation took us through the whole biopsy process.

I will forever be grateful that my doctor woke up on the right side of the bed and her Spidey senses tingled when she saw my films. I am sure she was on the fence, but what would it hurt to biopsy? What would it hurt to get this peace of mind? The doctor who ordered the biopsy *saved my life*! I later made the two doctors and the MRI tech the largest batch of "thank you for saving my life" cookies!

My GP, the doctor that gave me the referral for the mammogram, called me first thing in the morning the next day. It was September 4, 2020; I have not forgotten and will never forget that day. He said that my biopsy had come back positive and that I had invasive ductal carcinoma. He said he was sorry, and he did not know much more, but he was referring me to a breast specialist (Dr. D) to get more information and my treatment plan.

My treatment plan? Yesterday I was talking about being punched about the face/breast with the doctor performing the biopsy, and today I am getting a call from my doctor about a referral to an oncological surgeon about my treatment plan. I instantly felt alone, abandoned, betrayed, confused, blindsided. *This cannot be right. I am too young. I have an eighteen-month-old baby.* The ladies at the hospital were right. They made a mistake at the pathology lab.

This is a mistake! Not me! Not now!

I called my doctor back about five more times over the course of the day. I had to have him tell me this information repeatedly. The first three calls, I could not even write. I just had to hear it and try to mentally soak up all the information that he had for me. It was not real. Before the third call, my doctor called in a light Xanax prescription to my pharmacy. He said I was going to need it, and he was correct. My head was always spinning. I had nothing but *more* questions that could not be answered by my current doctor, and I did not *dare* Google *anything*. There is no way this could be real. I do not feel sick. I just got back from an hour-long jog. I do not have a lump; I do not have any of the symptoms that are common with a breast cancer diagnosis. That is when I realized that I needed to share my story and make sure that people know that cancer does not see age and does not have to conform to any rules.

In my opinion the worst thing in the world is waking up dead.

The next worst thing is to be told you have cancer.

I called the breast specialist / surgeon that I was referred to, and they initially told me that they were going to be able to see me in two weeks. Another gut punch. How can you know what I am going through and not get me in ASAP? I am lost, confused, and scared. I let the receptionist know that my time was worth nothing and that come Monday I would be sitting either in the parking lot or the waiting room to wait for an appointment or cancellation. I would be helping dust, cleaning pens, hell, I would even be vacuuming the waiting room, but I would not be sitting idly by while I had a cancer growing inside of me! Call it divine intervention, a cancellation, and/or professional persistence, but I ended up getting in for an appointment less than a week later.

I did not know how I was going to get through the weekend before my appointment. I did not sleep well. I do not do well with unanswered questions. I woke up at 4:00 a.m. every day. I took that opportunity to clean and try to clear my head, and I started writing. The morning of the appointment was the first time I wrote anything, and I wrote a letter to my son:

9.10.20, 4:35 a.m.

A letter to my son.

I got a mammogram to stay on top of my health. I do this for you, your father, and myself.

The mammogram/biopsy returned cancerous results.

It turns out to be invasive ductal carcinoma.

Today I am going with your grandmother to get that looked at and see what stage my cancer is and get a treatment plan.

I am scared. I am shocked. This is the unknown.

Now it is 6am, and it could be, and I am hoping, stage zero.

While I am already exhausted mentally, I know I need to fight more and harder. For you. For us. For our family. I never thought I would be in this position. Well, especially not this early. I am thirty-four, and you are just eighteen months old.

This is not fair to you. You deserve a healthy mother. A healthy family. One that can keep up with you. Challenge you. Have fun with you. A family that can give you the happiest childhood and the best life.

So that is why I am doing this. Everything I do, I do for you now. You are so many things, Chip. Already so dynamic with a killer personality at just 18 months old, and I cannot wait to watch you grow up.

So, in being as selfless as humanly possible, this has led to early detection, so for that I say thank you.

I want to write this letter on the unknowing side of my diagnosis because the only thing that will not change after these appointments today will be my unwavering and undying love for you and your father. You have made my life worth living. I am not finished.

I do not know where I will find the strength to fight, but I must.

Let us all send up prayers for a stage zero diagnosis and keep this moving.

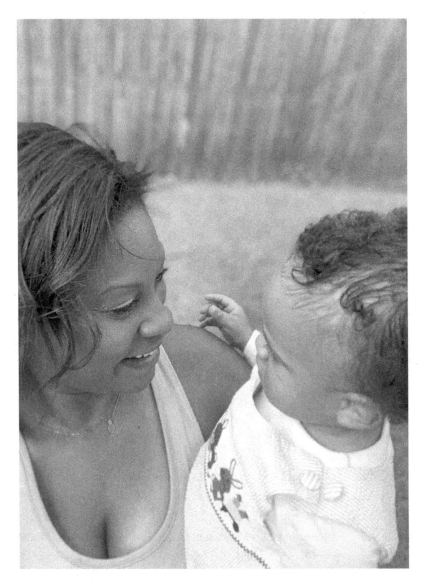

"You are my sun, my moon, and all my stars." E.E. Cummings

My best friend, Ebony, and I decided to make a Zoom call so she, my husband, and my sister could be present, I would have the recording to refer to, and we could all get the information at the same time. To this day I still have not gone back and listened to this recording. My mom came to my appointment with me. I wanted her there, and I also needed my family's medical history. I did not have all the details, and I wanted to be as informative as possible so I could get the best treatment.

That appointment was full of tears, exclusively from me. I realize now that I was grieving; that is officially when the grieving started. Until that appointment I was in limbo. I had not been staged, and I did not know what I was facing. Lauren BC (before cancer) died on September 4, and I was a new, different Lauren. Unknowingly I had entered preservation mode.

My first appointment, with the first oncological surgeon, I was bawling my eyes out. The woman started off telling me that I had stage one and we were going to start with chemo. None of that made sense to me. And she said it in a tone like "It does not have to make sense to you. I am the doctor, and you have cancer."

And I responded while crying in a tone like, "Well, I have googled a few things; those two things do not sound the same, and you are a bitch."

That appointment was long. It was around two hours. The doctor was thorough and told me a lot about breast cancer and what would and could happen from this point forward. I was told that I was a stage one and I needed to do genetic testing and have a lymph node biopsy that day. Of all the bad and scary things this first doctor told me that day, when I look back, I am surprised that she did not tell me more about the genetic test. If you are BRCA1 or BRCA2 positive, that has different implications, potentially additional surgeries, and your genetic test helps map your treatment plan.

The name "BRCA" is an abbreviation for "BReast CAncer gene." BRCA1 and BRCA2 are two different genes that have been found to impact a person's chances of developing breast cancer. Every human has both the BRCA1 and BRCA2 genes. Despite what their names might suggest, BRCA genes do not cause breast cancer. In fact, these genes normally play a big role in preventing breast cancer. They help repair DNA breaks that can lead to cancer and the uncontrolled growth of tumors. Because of this, the BRCA genes are known as tumor suppressor genes.

However, sometimes tumor suppression genes do not work properly. When a gene becomes altered or broken, it does not function correctly. This is called a gene mutation. It is estimated that one in eight women, or approximately 12 percent, will be diagnosed with breast cancer in her lifetime. Women with certain genetic mutations have a higher lifetime risk of the disease.

Women with a BRCA1 or BRCA2 mutations who overcome their breast cancer with treatment appear to have a higher-than-average chance of developing a second cancer. This is called a recurrence. Cancers related to a BRCA1 mutation are also more likely to be triple negative breast cancer, which can be more aggressive and difficult to treat.

There are also other gene mutations besides BRCA that could increase the risk of breast cancer. The most prominent of these is PALB2. As with BRCA1 and BRCA2, testing for other genetic mutations is recommended only if you are at high risk for that particular gene. (National Breast Cancer Foundation 2020)

One of the last things that the doctor told me that day was that my breast cancer (HER2-positive breast cancer) "likes to hang out in the brain" and "if there is cancer present in your lymph nodes, there will need to be a different conversation."

This is a lot for anyone to digest, especially all at once. Spoiler alert: we had to have that different conversation.

9.12.20

On September 10 I had a biopsy on my lymph nodes, and that came back positive. So now this week I will require the MRI and PET to determine the size of my breast lesion and to make sure it has not spread. There is no lump on my breast. The calcifications are under the breast and far from the nipple. Hard to find by the doctor and difficult to find on ultrasound to biopsy.

My mind is blown.

My heart is shattered.

I am terrified.

I have never been this scared of anything-the unknown of the PET.

After my lymph nodes came back cancerous, the doctor called me and told me that I now had to have an MRI, a PET scan, and a CT of my brain and body to determine if the cancer had spread and to determine if I was treatable or curable. At this point I just *lost it*; I just spent the rest of the day crying. After hours of appointments the day before, now you are calling me to tell me of all the referrals you have sent in for tests to redetermine what stage I am in.

Over the next ten days, I had an MRI on my brain, a PET scan on my body, a CT on my chest, and an echo on my heart. It was stressful, but I used humor to take the edge off. Well, that and Xanax.

> A positron emission tomography (PET) scan is an imaging test that allows your doctor to check for diseases in your body. The scan uses a special dye containing radioactive tracers. These tracers are either swallowed, inhaled, or injected into a vein in your arm, depending on what part of the body is being examined. Certain organs and tissues then absorb the tracer.
>
> When detected by a PET scanner, the tracers help your doctor to see how well your organs and tissues are working. The tracer will collect in areas of higher chemical activity, which is helpful because certain tissues of the body, and certain diseases, have a higher level of chemical activity. These areas of disease will show up as bright spots on the PET scan. (Healthline.com 2018)

I try to laugh or find the humor in everything. The funniest part of the diagnostic testing was the PET scan. It is a serious test, but once you are in the cancer seat, everything is what it is until you get the results. It is a Schrodinger's cat situation, and I guess I am the cat in the box, and I am both alive and dead. I get in the room, and the nurse tells me that I *must* relax, or the tracer will not do its job. I turn on my music, and she takes my phone. She opens a lead box, and there is a lead needle inside. It hits the table with a *loud* metallic clank/thud. It is glowing. Like in the opening scene from *The Simpsons*. I know that it is nuclear, but it was that color.

She injects me *and then* tells me that I will be radioactive for the next twenty-four hours. Um, *what?* I already knew that, but shouldn't you tell me this *beforehand* so I can prepare? My son had to stay with the grandparents for the night because you cannot be around children while you are *radioactive*. What the what?

I did check to see if I glowed in the dark, and unfortunately, I did not.

The results of my scans concluded that my cancer had not spread further than my lymph nodes and it was not in my brain.

Hallelujah!

At the appointment, the doctor told me we would start with chemo and that I would be starting chemo in three weeks. That blew my socks off, and I do not even wear socks! She did not have the results from the lymph node biopsy or my scans. WTF. She mentioned that I would be getting a shot every month that would put my ovaries to sleep so as to protect them from the chemo. Putting them to sleep for a year sounded better than a medically induced menopause, but marketing aside, the fact remains—*medically induced menopause*. It comes with all the consolation prizes of menopause you have seen and heard, and hot flashes are real. The devil is a lie. *Do not believe him*; remember that apple thing with Eve? *Not cool!*

There was not a ton of research and data available for me on my reproductive health. I am not done having children yet, and I was not going to allow cancer to take that from me as well.

9.25.20

Yesterday I had four appointments. I think that is the last day I will have so many. I had:

- A COVID test for the chemo port surgery. *Do not let anyone tell you they're not that bad.* That nurse was able to find the memory of my sixth birthday, scramble it around and rip it out through my nose.

- My follow-up IVF appt to get and start my drugs

- My final appt with my oncologist before I begin chemo with forms staging and diagnosis

- And I had an echocardiogram on my heart because chemo causes reversible heart damage.

My oncologist, who looks like Nev from Catfish, is so thorough and clear that he has made cancer not sad or scary really. I have not cried in his office once!

I have since replaced the first doctor, and I am elated with my new surgeon. One of the most important things that I want to convey is that you and your doctors should be working together. You have the right to a second or third opinion. If you do not vibe with your surgeon or your doctor, replace them. I am referring to any instance, not just cancer. You need to be able to rely on, confide in, and be honest with your doctor. Also, if you feel that your doctor does not listen to you or address all of your concerns, that is a problem too. You know your body best, and if you have a concern, your doctor should be as concerned as you are. If you are in a situation where you do not feel comfortable with your doctor, call your insurance provider, and get a list of providers that are covered.

After all the testing and the results came back, in September 2020, I was officially diagnosed with stage 2 HER2-positive hormone receptor negative BRCA negative invasive ductal carcinoma (a.k.a. IDC) at the age of thirty-four. I called my support village and let them know about my diagnosis and what I had gone through from July to September. I also begged people to get checked and start the process. I just do not want anyone to feel the way I felt that day. I just really hope I can forget that pain with time.

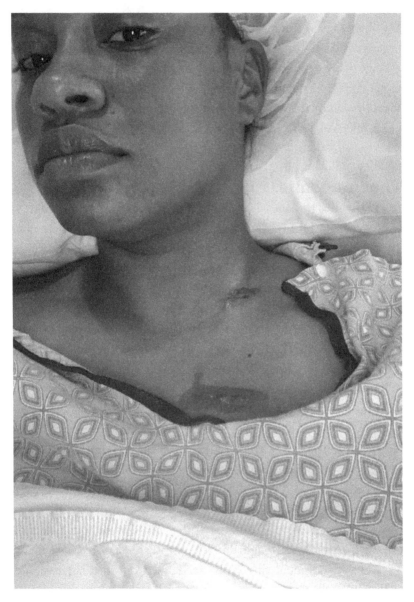

Post-port surgery

My chances of getting breast cancer before the age of seventy with a negative BRCA number and my genetics was 12 percent, and the percentage of breast cancer patients diagnosed with HER2-positive while at the same time being HR-negative is 5 percent. I guess I should play the lottery and look out for lightning a little more. In the middle of a pandemic. Yes, I did say "pandemic."

The Pandemic

"COVID-19 is the disease caused by a new coronavirus called SARS-CoV-2. The WHO first learned of this new virus on 31 December 2019, following a report of a cluster of cases of 'viral pneumonia' in Wuhan, People's Republic of China" (WHO 2020).

"The COVID-19 pandemic, also known as the coronavirus pandemic, is an ongoing global pandemic of coronavirus disease 2019 (COVID-19) caused by severe acute respiratory syndrome coronavirus 2 (SARS-CoV-2). The virus was first identified in December 2019 in Wuhan, China. The World Health Organization declared a Public Health Emergency of International Concern regarding COVID-19 on 30 January 2020, and later declared a pandemic on 11 March 2020. As of 12 April 2021, more than 136 million cases have been confirmed, with more than 2.93 million deaths attributed to COVID-19, making it one of the deadliest pandemics in history" (Wikipedia 2020).

The pandemic made this cancer diagnosis a bit more difficult as I was not always allowed a visitor with me to doctor appointments. Cancer is a lot to go through, and you already feel isolated in so many ways. To literally and physically be isolated during diagnosis and treatment took it to a whole other level. There were certain doctor appointments that I had to go to alone, and I had to do chemo alone. That was probably the hardest and saddest part of all of this.

Type A Questions to Ask at Your Initial Appointment

(Make sure to bring a pen and paper.)

- Are you an oncologist or an oncological surgeon? (If the doctor is an oncological surgeon, will you also need an oncologist?)

- What kind of cancer do I have?

- Has it spread?

- Is it local?

- Is it in my lymph nodes?

- What am I being staged at?

- What other tests do I need?

  - CT scan
  - genetic testing
  - MRI
  - echocardiogram
  - PET scan

- What is my treatment plan?

- How aggressive is my cancer?

- How will any of these treatments affect my fertility?

- What is my prognosis?

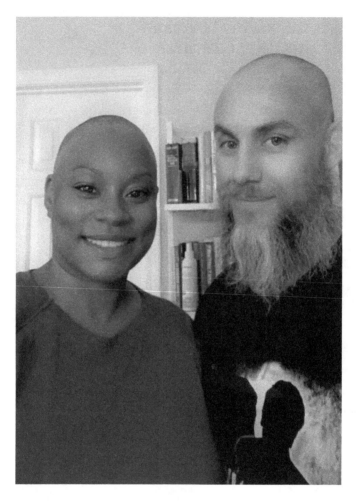

"My lobster!"

CHAPTER 4:

Caregivers

You are going to need caretaker(s) and a group of people that you can depend on while you are going through treatment. It is a lot to deal with mentally, physically, and emotionally! I know that everyone does not have the same family set up, logistical or otherwise, but you need to find your people. Just as you need to find a medical team that works for you, you will need your people. If you live alone, reach out to others in the cancer community (locally or online), and that will at least get you started mentally and emotionally.

In my village I have, first and foremost, my husband and partner in life and my family (my mom, dad, and sister), and they are my rocks. I also have the most supportive in-laws.

Another integral part of my village is my best friend, Dr. Ebony Jade Hilton. She is the kindest, most beautiful human alive, as well as being supersmart and funny. So, back to how she is in my village. Not everyone has a doctor as a best friend. Ebony was researching all the things my doctors were saying, helping me understand any clinical speak I did not initially understand and helping me weigh outcomes of decisions I had to make.

Additionally, in my village I have quite a few cancer survivors and a nurse that have been beacons for me—Emily, Rebecca, and Kirby, I cannot thank you enough.

I just cannot say enough about my village and how they have kept me grounded, organized, and focused. This may not be something that crosses your mind, but your support system "village" may not know how best to support you. Just because you are family, you may not be speaking the same love languages. There is also a lot to do during treatment, so they may have forgotten something you said in passing a week or two ago. Please just remember who is there for you and showing up when you need them.

My village is made up mostly of family and people who have been through this, but I found a lot of people that I trust and can confide in on Instagram. The cancer community on Instagram has been the most pleasant surprise. Everyone responds quickly, and if they cannot find an answer for you, they will try to find it for you. Which is to say, even if your family does not live close to you, *you are not alone.* There are services that can drive you to and from treatment and free group therapy. I honestly feel that I talk to my online support groups more about my cancer than my village at times. I never want to be a burden or scare my friends and family with my thoughts, but there is nothing like the understating and symbiosis that comes from talking to someone who is going through what you're going through when you're going through it.

1.28.21

I have never asked why. I have asked who, what, when, where, and how, but never why. I just took it on the chin and kept it moving. When I look at old pictures, I'm in disbelief at my old life. I'm not in disbelief that I had cancer. I am in disbelief—and don't say often enough—that

I am cancer-free, but to be honest I'm almost more shocked that I wake up every day and keep going through my new normal versus just completely breaking down. I am on the verge often of crying. At times I give in. It makes me feel better. Sometimes I push it deep down, and that doesn't make me feel better. I do it to make the people around me feel better or more comfortable. I just often think about and have to pull from the strength of my ancestors and angels, whom I know that are around me and a source of my strength; I have to call on them. I try to give them my angst or call on them to help me process these overwhelming and encompassing feelings, thoughts, and shortcomings.

Being a caregiver at times is as hard as being the patient. Caregivers love you, do not want this for you, and at times feel helpless. They may even take on some of the symptoms that you have—fatigue, headaches, exhaustion, stress, hopelessness, depression. Just remember that you are not a burden; cancer is the burden. The people that are present want to be around and want to help you. The most important thing is mental health and knowing your limits, and that goes for the patient as well as the caregiver. You also will want to make sure to be as clear and communicative as you can. Unfortunately, none of us can read minds, so you need to talk about your needs and whether or not they are being met. There is a lot of help out, there and not one person can do it *all*!

Type A Questions to Ask Your Potential Caretaker

- Are you in a good emotional, mental, and physical place to take on being a caretaker?

- What is the plan for the children (if applicable)?

- Do you have reliable transportation?

- Will you take leave from work or try to keep working?

- Do you have a flexible schedule? (If not, look into FMLA or what your job offers for caretaker leave.)

Type A Tips for Having a Successful Relationship with Your Caretaker(s)

- Be gentle; it is a hard time for everyone involved.

- Remember, your caretaker has their own life too.

- Meditate, together or separately.

- Seek therapy—group, couple, or solo.

- Plan enjoyable things to do together, not just things surrounding cancer and care.

- Write everything down.

- Look for additional help to relieve your caretaker.

- Prepping meals or buying prepared meals saves time and energy for later.

- If possible, have a schedule to stick to so everyone has clear expectations.

- Communicate your gratitude.

Type A Tips for Good Gifts to Give Someone Who is Newly Diagnosed

- Comfortable socks

- Candles

- Chapstick

- A nice blanket

- Soft button-up pajamas (very helpful after surgery)

- Lotions—chemo and radiation dry you out

- Metal cups or water bottles to promote hydration

- Chemo shirt

- Gift cards for food delivery or dropping off food

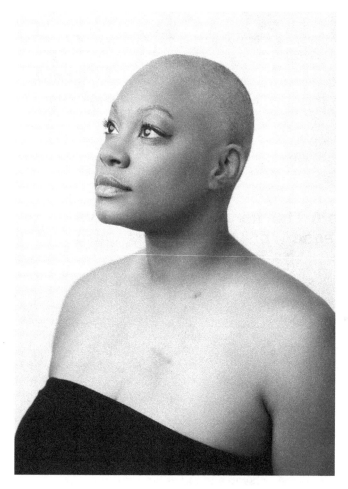

"Looking towards the future" By Jody Mack

CHAPTER 5:

IVF

The oversights in care due to the AYA cancer community being under served are most apparent in reproductive and fertility conversations. It is reported that approximately 41 percent of AYA cancer patients are consulted about their reproductive health and futures. This may be because of the age range that this group is comprised of. It is difficult to think about what you want for your life and to make a definitive decision about children when you are sixteen years old. Another very real obstacle is the cost of fertility preservation. You will want to check with your insurance company to see if any or all of the cost of treatment is covered. "As of August 2020, 19 states have passed fertility insurance coverage laws, 13 of those laws include IVF coverage, and 10 states have fertility preservation laws for iatrogenic (medically induced) infertility" (What Are My Options? 2020).

"In vitro fertilization (IVF) is a complex series of procedures used to help with fertility. During IVF, mature eggs are collected (retrieved) from ovaries and fertilized by sperm in a lab. Then the fertilized egg (embryo) or eggs (embryos) are transferred to a uterus. One full cycle of IVF takes about three weeks. Sometimes these steps are split into different parts and the process can take longer. IVF is the most effective form of assisted reproductive technology. The procedure can be done using your own eggs and your partner's sperm. Or IVF may involve eggs, sperm or embryos from a known or anonymous donor" (Mayo Clinic 2019).

In my case nothing was covered, and that is where the assistance from Livestrong Foundation came in. They covered all the initial drugs for an egg retrieval and had preset costs that they had negotiated with a selection of fertility clinics. One thing that I did not expect was for everything to be a la carte. You pay for the preliminary drugs, the blood work, the visits, the anesthesia for the egg retrieval, the egg retrieval procedure, genetic testing, storage, as well as implantation and the drugs for implantation when the time comes, all separately.

"According to the N.C.S.L., the average I.V.F. cycle can cost anywhere from $12,000 to $17,000 (not including medication). With medication, the cost can rise to closer to $25,000" (Klein 2020).

This is a substantial amount of money for anyone, but this is also an added stress on top of a cancer diagnosis when you have no idea what this disease is going to cost you, financially, in the end. It is recommended that you ask for a referral to an endocrinologist / reproductive specialist for a consult within twenty-four hours of a cancer diagnosis. This is so that your oncologist and your endocrinologist have time to talk about your diagnosis, your treatment plan, and determine if you have enough time for fertility preservation before you begin treatment. That is a huge ask when you have just been given life-changing information and then have made major decisions. This is all just proactive. There is a high chance that your fertility will not be affected by your treatment, depending on the kind of cancer that you have and your treatment plan. In the unfortunate case that it is, there are other options; do not forget about adoption, surrogacy, donor eggs, and donor sperm.

As a side note, one of my breasties was told at her consultation that eggs last three to five years but embryos do not have a shelf life. That may be helpful in your decision about whether to freeze eggs or embryos, even though the cost will differ between the two. Thank you, Parrish!

We did not have long to decide whether to do a cycle of IVF. I had one day to decide, and that also meant that I would have to push back treatment, but only by a week. I did not know what to do. My husband left the decision up to me, but he was for it. My mom was for it; my sister was for it. By happenstance, Dr. D called me that day. I was on my way to take my sister out for dinner for her birthday. It was three days shy of a month from my initial diagnosis. I will never forget the conversation.

Dr. D said, "Lauren, you're a beautiful, *young* thirty-four-year-old woman with an aggressive form of cancer"

I thought, *Um, you have barely seen me with my mask off!* I said, "I am just looking for answers and guidance." I am a very decisive person, but I need help. I need people who want to lay out my options.

"Yes, Lauren, you are a beautiful, young, healthy"—*Um, I have cancer*, I thought to myself—"thirty-four-year-old mother with a young child, and we just want to let you know what all your options are. It is rare to have a patient like you."

That was one of the last conversations we had because not all the conversations with her were that helpful. Though I did not care for the Dr. D and I was in the process of replacing her, she was the deciding factor in deciding to postpone chemo for one week to complete one round of IVF. So, for that, *and only that*, I thank her.

My mom later asked me if I did not like her because she delivered all the bad news. That is not why I did not care for her. It was her bedside manner. You know if you vibe with someone. We did not vibe, but I do appreciate her taking off her doctor hat *one time* to help me decide whether or not to do IVF.

10.01.20

We have begun IVF, and I will be thirty-five in eighteen days, and even though I know that your fertility does not "fall off of a cliff" at thirty-five, I also know that the terrain gets a little rougher around that age. For my diagnosis, stage 2 HER2-positive breast cancer, I will need to go on a cocktail of four chemo drugs for six cycles and take one drug for an additional eight months. I must have at least a solo mastectomy and radiation for the cancer that has spread to my lymph nodes. They also want me to put a pin in any procreation for a year after treatment is finished. My doctors already know I have a type A personality, and most of them love it. I track my vitals at home and come to appointments with written notes and questions and all the forms I need for insurance and work. Others do not care for it. They respond to me as if I have googled everything before I show up and am telling them how to do to their job. I have been careful not to do this. So, to the doctors who do not appreciate it, first, you are fired. You are just not that into me, and same here. Second, we must be our own advocates for health care. I have made this my mantra especially because I am a young black woman in America. The doctors that did not like my level of organization are now gone. They are not part of my treatment team or my healing village. Your energy was off, and I rebuke you.

I woke up again at 4:00 a.m., and I felt weird. Why would I not feel weird? I have had my chemo port surgery; my chest constantly hurts. My first surgery with cancer was getting the port for chemo. A port is a small plastic or metal disk that they insert under the skin in your upper chest. It is how you receive your chemo treatments or how they draw your blood, which they do very often. My port surgery was *weird*. I was out, but I was awake. It is like Lasik. You need to be awake so you can turn your head and they can make sure that it is functioning, but they are also cutting into your neck and chest, and you do not feel anything. Very wild experience.

I now have a nineteen-month-old, and every morning is like *50 First Dates*.

I must constantly remind myself that I have cancer—you know, because I have not started chemo and I still have my hair. I have to remember what has to get done today for myself, my self-care, my *baby*, my husband, my household, and my health, which is now a separate entity from myself and my self-care.

Every morning I wake up and I feel good, but then I must remember that I have cancer.

Then I remember where I am and where I am in my journey—*not even a month, dammit*. Ok, I can do this. I wake up with my period. My first thought is "This is not right because we are on a cycle of IVF, and is this not *another* drug that is supposed to stop your period so they can bulk up your eggs, so they are big enough to steal out of your hen house?" I thought I had just seen all my hard work and money flushed down the toilet!

After playing Candy Crush and watching the clock to the second to wait for a "normal" hour to call the fertility doc on her *cell* (7:01 a.m.), I call her, and she is not *too* worried. We are not implanting now, and we have not triggered the eggs into the follicles that we are *pumping* up. Ok, so I am choosing to trust her, but I do not ever believe *anyone* until I see it with my own eyes. Since we are four days (*hopefully*) from retrieval, I have a blood test and ultrasound this morning to make sure what she said was correct. I do not have another month do to this again. I start chemo in *one* week. I understand that I am lucky that my decision to push chemo was only affected by one week, but if this does not work, I still have to pay *her*!

IVF was not as bad as I thought it would be. I have helped friends with their shots before and watched acquaintances go through the process, and I have heard it all! I didn't gain any weight, and usually if I look at a salad with dressing on it, I grow another chin instantly. I do not believe I was any more moody than normal, but you would have to ask my husband about that part. In my opinion the hardest part of doing IVF is purposely sticking and injecting yourself with hormones so that you can do all you can do to try to have another baby after all of this *while* your first child is going through toddler teething and acting a donkey *all* over the house. You question a lot of your life choices. Now that Chip is officially into his "terrible twos," I often think about calling the facility where the popsicle babies are and telling them to unplug the freezer. I *joke*, but for real, though, can I get a *break*? It also does not help when you are trying to psych yourself up to stab yourself in the stomach and your baby is begging for medicine too. Just imagine. That part was cute; he melts me.

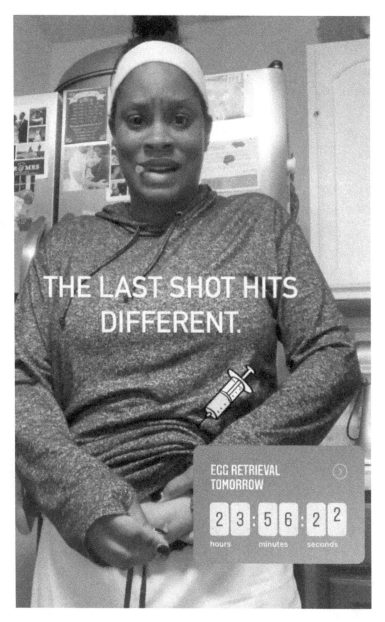

Lupron trigger shot before egg retrieval

Livestrong helped us a lot with the freezing of our embryos. If you are newly diagnosed or looking into fertility preservation, investigate the assistance that the Livestrong Foundation provides. They sent us all the drugs that we needed; I was in disbelief.

10.2.20

I am waiting on my egg retrieval, and the final countdown for my first chemo infusion has begun. I feel at peace a bit. I know that sounds funky but follow. I have made all the jokes and plans that I can to make everyone around me feel as comfortable as they can be. I will transition my hair to a shorter length, I will dye it wild colors, and I will wear cutting-edge wigs. I do not want anyone to know that I am scared shitless, scared of the unknown. I am thirty-four, and that is not terribly young, but I am damn sure not old. I am trying to think positively, but what if it comes back? What if chemo hurts? The only thing I have never wanted in my life is to hurt my mother, father, sister, husband, and son, and I feel like I have deflated and disappointed them all with one blow.

10.6.20

I am very much excited about the egg retrieval and oddly excited to start chemo. I am scared. Very scared. I am looking forward to starting chemo because I have already had the scan that tells me I do not have cancer anywhere else in my body, and I want to kill the cancer that is there now. I yearn to get better. I feel awesome. I just feel like a run-of-the-mill thirty-four-year-old with an eighteen-month-old. So, a little achy and at times inexplicably hungover when I have not even had a drink, but I feel great. That is what is so weird about my cancer. I do not feel bad. And now all these experts and people that I am to trust with my life are telling me that I will need poison in my body that will make me feel like shit to be healthy. It is a true mind-bender when you think about it.

One month from diagnosis, I had my egg retrieval. I only felt real discomfort on the morning of the procedure. The shots did not bother me; the nearly daily check-ins, blood work, and transvaginal ultrasounds did not bother me. But the morning of the retrieval, I was nearly as bloated as the day I gave birth. Things went well, and that was a fun distraction.

I had never thought negatively about IVF, other than the price tag; to be honest I had never really thought about IVF. But there are people who do not get a lot of eggs or embryos. I never thought of that as a possibility. But remember it only takes *one*. One fertilized egg for a baby. No matter how many they get from you, just remember it only takes one.

During this process, especially during IVF, I wondered often if it would have been better to have children before or after cancer. There are pros and cons to both sides. I think that is why I felt so uncomfortable at the fertility clinic pre-chemo. I had a baby, and I felt like I was somewhere I was not supposed to be, learning, and seeing things I was not supposed to know.

I am beyond grateful and blessed to have our son Chip, and that took a lot of pressure off of my heart worrying about future children. We would have been heartbroken to have not had the choice or opportunity to have another baby. IVF took another load off my back and heart. So, we did all we could before I started treatment. But then if you already have a small child while you are going through treatment, it makes it harder. When you have children, you are no longer on your own schedule. You are on theirs, so that makes recovering a little harder. I could not control when I needed to sleep or run to the restroom. That is just another way that my husband was beyond helpful. These are things that more and more cancer patients have to consider these days as women are diagnosed earlier and earlier in life.

One night I was trying to get him to go to be after a sleep regression and daylight saving. We were on a beach get away and I put Chip in our bed to try to get him more tired. I whispered I love you and he whispered it back. That is s one of my favorite things that he does; when he whispers what I whispered to him back to me. He put his tiny hand on my cheek and asked me why I had water in my eyes. I was crying because that's one of my favorite moments and it will become one of my favorite memories. It's quiet. It's dark. We are making eye contact and his tiny hand is on my cheek. There's no tantrum, there is no back talk. It's like he's looking into my soul and knows I need comfort and peace. He is that empathetic and intuitive at two years old. He is my everything. I think I found my answer. For me it's easier with my boy. Maybe it's easy with one baby. To see what you're fighting for. I am fighting for him. I do everything for my Carl's. Not myself. Just them. They do everything for me and I am fighting for my life for them.

One of the scariest things I have heard about is women finding out about their cancer during pregnancy, and my heart just breaks for these warriors. Cancer is hard. Being a parent is hard. Being pregnant is hard. Combining all of those things—that pressure just turn these women into diamonds.

The very next day, I began chemo.

Type A Questions to Ask Your Oncologist about Fertility

- Has my cancer affected my fertility? Will it affect my fertility?

- Does my treatment plan have any known adverse effects on fertility?

- Do you have any breakdowns of studies that might be helpful?

- Do I have time for fertility preservation before I start treatment?

- Do I have time for more than one cycle, if needed?

- Do you have an endocrinologist that you work with or that you can refer me to?

Type A Questions to Ask your Fertility Specialist

- What will genetic testing tell us?

- Should I preserve eggs or embryos?

- Can you only perform genetic testing on embryos? Can you test on eggs and sperm solo?

- What are my options for embryos or eggs that we do not implant?

- How many can I implant at a time?

- What is my projected success rate for a live birth?

- Do you have payment plans or inhouse grants for fertility cost assistance?

- Can you please check my health insurance to see if any of this is covered?

Type A Tips for IVF

- Stay hydrated

- Eat a healthy and balanced diet

- Take time off where needed. This is a stressful time, and the procedure can be affected by stress.

- No smoking

- No drinking

- Take your vitamins

- Get good quality sleep

CHAPTER 6:

Racial Disparities in Medicine

In case you do not know by now, I am an African American woman. That is not an easy thing to be these days, nor has it ever really been so in our country's history.

I am a black woman.

I am a black mother.

I am a black patient.

I am a woman who works in technology.

I am a woman who likes sports.

I am a minority everywhere I go, and before that did not bother me, but I am on an island. And island with people that I chose or who chose me but on which there are few who look like me.

This is not about race; this is about strength. All my life I have been told that I am strong and resilient. I tell people I have cancer and because I do not cry right then and there, they say, "You are so strong; you are going to get through this. No problem."

I feel like that is like telling me I am supposed to be a good singer (which I *am not*) or a good athlete because I am black. Just because, out of necessity, I have built these brick walls, *multiple* walls, to protect my heart and sense of self and my humanity and my family against the world for the last thirty-four years does not really mean I am strong. It just means I am a warrior turned survivor. I am saving my strength for my parents. It worries me to worry them. I did *enough* of that in my twenties. I have been trying to clean up my act or the last near-decade, and *now this*! I do not want them to see their firstborn bald and frail.

The most selfish thing I can say now is that I am glad this is happening while I am young, so I have my mommy and all of the strength I am going to have. Others are not so lucky, and I recognize that every day.

So yes, I am strong, but I feel that people are going through their own five stages of grief and justifying it happening to me—not out of schadenfreude or anything but justifying it because I am the strongest person they know, so I was put up as tribute. Well Mockingjay this, cancer. I often feel that when I tell people I have breast cancer, or *had* breast cancer, they repeat the stat in their head, "one in eight women," then they count how many women are around. Um, just as a heads-up, cancer patient do not like it. We already have cancer. You do not have to reinforce the statistics.

I know you have seen the pictures, experienced it, or known someone who has gone through it. But everyone looks different while in treatment. In the middle of my treatment, literally after my fourth chemo cycle, I did a photo shoot to show exactly that. That everyone looks different during treatment. I was a little tired, and I did have to wipe a bloody nose in between some of the shots, but we kept on. As for the nosebleeds, I am still having to magic eraser blood off of the walls from where I sneezed and did not know where the blood landed. It is the worst "hunt" I have ever been on.

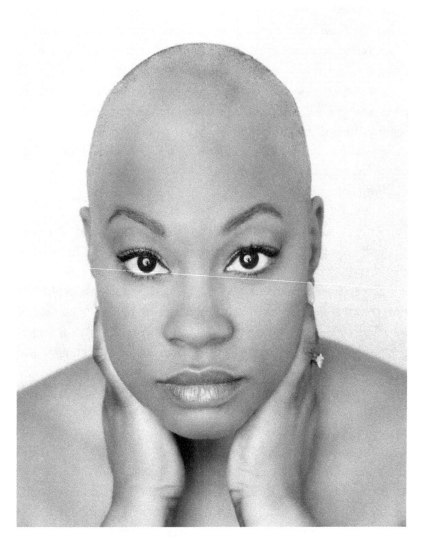

"Just Me" taken by Jody Mack

As regards cancer disparities in the black community:

African Americans have a higher cancer burden and face greater obstacles to cancer prevention, detection, treatment, and survival. In fact, Black people have the highest death rate and shortest survival of any racial/ethnic group for most cancers in the U.S. Research has shown that:

African Americans experience more illness, worse outcomes, and premature death compared to whites.

African Americans have the highest death rate and shortest survival of any racial/ethnic group for most cancers. African American men also have the highest cancer incidence.

Cancer death rates in black men is twice as high as in Asians and Pacific Islanders, who have the lowest rates.

Prostate cancer death rates in black men are more than double those of every other racial/ethnic group.

Black women are 40% more likely to die of breast cancer than white women and are twice as likely to die if they are over 50.

About a third of African American women reported experiencing racial discrimination at a health provider visit.

Living in segregated communities and areas highly populated with African Americans has been associated with increased chances of getting diagnosed with cancer after it has spread, along with having higher death rates and lower rates of survival from breast and lung cancers. (Cancer Disparities in the Black Community 2020)

10.7.21

I personally have not experienced any overt racism or discrimination in my interactions with medical professionals, lately, but I am very outspoken about the level of care that I give myself and expect from my health care provider. I have wondered when my husband and I go to the doctor together, Am I going to be taken more or less seriously because he is a white man? Am I enough, on my own, for this doctor to care about me?

While I was being interviewed for *But Seriously: The Cancer Podcast*, the host, Bert Scholl, a two-time cancer survivor, gave me some really good advice that he uses himself, "I ask the doctors if I can call them by their first name!" I had never thought of that. I usually just call them doc, but that is a great icebreaker and can help to bridge a relationship! Or you could be like me and want, so badly, for people to feel comfortable around you, despite the cancer, that you tell self-deprecating jokes and act inappropriate and/or awkward in social settings.

Type A Tips for Building a Rapport with Your Doctors and Specialists

- If you are comfortable doing so, ask your doctor if you can call them by their first name.

- If you do not understand what your doctor is saying, ask as many questions as necessary.

- If you do not understand the clinical speak, they are using, ask them to use different terminology.

- Be honest with your doctor; they cannot best assist you if they do not have the whole story.

- Be prepared for your appointments with questions and concerns written down and have a pen and paper to write down the responses.

CHAPTER 7:

Grants

The Livestrong Foundation was the gateway for me to learn about grants and how they can help so much. I work loosely around grants, and honestly, I thought they were mainly B2B (business to business). But after working with Livestrong and seeing how easy and friendly they were, I was interested in seeing whether there were other grants that could assist me with the financial aspect of my diagnosis. Grants can help cancer patients with anything from childcare costs to airfare to treatments, gas, medical bills, groceries, and so on. Below are the organizations that I have received assistance from (so far), but please do your research and get all the help that you can. Some foundations are cancer or disease specific, others are geographically specific, and some are based on income. Grants are so important because this money can help level the playing field for cancer patients whose lives will be disproportionally affected by these costs. Below are some of the organizations that awarded grants to me. I honestly found them through assistance with my nurse navigator, Google, and Instagram.

Livestrong Foundation

United Breast Care Foundation

The Atrium Foundation

Pink Shoes Inc.

Fighting Pretty

Susan G. Komen

The Boon Project

Living Beyond Breast Cancer

Tigerlily Foundation

One Day to Remember

Cleaning for a Reason

Sisters Network Inc.

Provision Project

BRCA Strong

Type A Tips for Grants

- A lot of foundations pay out grants until they are out of resources for the quarter or their determined period, so you will want to apply for grants as soon as you see the application.

- There are some grants that only support certain areas, counties, and/or states, so make sure to read the fine print so as not to waste time.

- Most applications require a letter from your doctor and/or a copy of your initial pathology reports to confirm your diagnosis.

- Most grants are paid directly to the creditor, so be ready to supply your utility or rent bill with the grant application.

- A lot of these foundations are smaller and have a set limit on how much they can and will assist, and that is usually noted in the application instructions.

- There are some grants that specifically pay for medical bills, but there are a lot more that pay for utilities, costs related to childcare, and other living expenses. This way you can reallocate the money that would have gone to living expenses to medical bills.

- Some applications will only be accepted if they are filled out and/or submitted by your nurse navigator or your hospital's social worker.

- You should meet them before treatment starts, but if you have not been introduced, ask your doctor or nurse for that contact information.

- Keep track of application submissions.

- Some foundations take upward of twelve weeks to process an application if it is not for an emergency fund grant. You will want to know your application status and have information to provide if you call or email for a status update.

- Not all applications have a submission confirmation page, so make sure to print your application (before submission) or take detailed notes on submitted applications.

CHAPTER 8:

Chemo

The first day of chemo is like the first day of school. You do not know how things work, the staff is *so* friendly, but the patients do not recognize you, and you do not know whom to talk to. Also, you are one of few people there with hair. They know you are a newbie; they can smell it on you. I felt so prepared. I had my chemo shirt, which Trey bought me. It unzips on both sides in front of your shoulders, so it does not matter which side your port is on, and it is very convenient for the nurse to access your port. It is one of the most thoughtful gifts that I received.

The first day of chemo was full of emotions, and I was on a learning curve. Before you begin chemo, you have chemo school. Chemo school was a bit overwhelming and shocking. They tell you what will and can happen and who to call in what instance. They tell you about side effects that you will and can have and what has happened to others. Chemo school is just like any other school or training—they give you the information, but there are things they gloss over or forget. They definitely did not go over the diarrhea part enough.

I had my chemo infusions at the hematology and oncology center, not at the hospital. I liked that better, personally. I think it helped with my anxiety toward treatment as I did not have to go to a large, confusing, overwhelming hospital. I get my blood drawn through my port, and then they flush my port. As a side note, I had a double port. It was recommended for me, and that is what was written up for me to have implanted during my surgery. I did not know anything about that at the time. I was glad to have had a double port. If one side is not clear, then you have another option. To flush a clogged port takes a lot, around another hour. I get to see my doctor while we wait on the blood results to see if I am healthy enough to get the drugs. My chemo sessions are around eight hours long, and because of the pandemic, you are not allowed visitors in the chemo suite.

The day went by quickly. I was still recovering from the egg retrieval the day before, and they give you Benadryl with your chemo cocktail, so you sleep a lot. It was relaxing; everyone was very accommodating, and then the day was gone. You do not feel the effects of the drugs right off because they give you steroids intravenously too. At the end of the first day, I also got my first Zoladex shot, and they put my Neulesta shot in my arm. Zoladex is very similar to Lupron, but there was a Lupron shortage, so I was prescribed Zoladex. These are ovary suppressing drugs that protect your ovaries from chemotherapy as they enter you into a medically induced menopause.

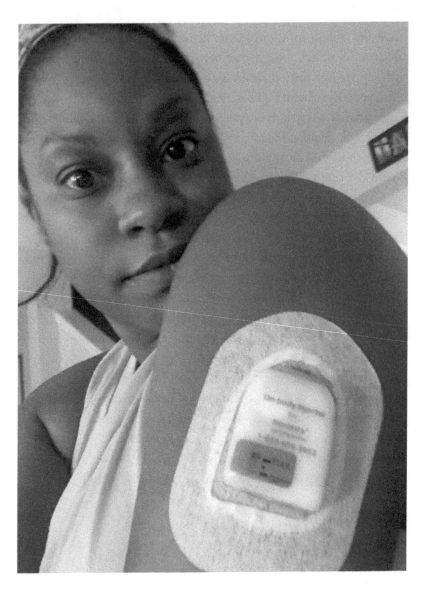

My first Nulesta device.

Neulesta is a necessary evil. It comes in a device they stick on your body, and twenty-four hours after chemo it administers a drug used to help your body make more white blood cells. White blood cells are important to help you fight off infections. Neulasta stimulates your immune system into producing more white blood cells. If you do not know (I did not), white blood cells are made in your bone marrow. Everyone gets pain in different places. They stuck that sucker on my arm, and as it activates, the small plastic needle pop outs and penetrates your skin. They say it feels like a rubber band snap. I was reminded of the biopsy doctor who said the next day I would feel like I was punched in the breast. It did not feel like a rubber band snap. It felt like a plastic needle being automatically shoved into nice little unsuspecting arm. This first shot I felt it in my pelvis and my spine. I could not walk without a lot of pain. I also was prescribed steroids for nausea that kept me from sleeping. I did not sleep for four days.

The fist chemo cycle and the days following were terrible. But I got through it, and I learned what worked for me. I would take ibuprofen for the Neulesta pain preventatively, I used a negative ion mat for full body recovery, and I got acupuncture and massage therapy to combat other aches and pains. I made sure to go on at least a thirty-minute walk daily and ate what I could when I could. I was very tired during chemo. I have never been that tired in my whole life, not even during pregnancy, and it was a different kind of tired. I would just pass out for hours. But that was for only about four days after treatment. Then the stomach problems would kick in. I was on a cycle every three weeks, so I would be worse for wear the first week. Second week was always stomach stuff (a.k.a. serious diarrhea, but at times I may just refer to that as stomach stuff), and the third week I was good. Just in time for another infusion.

I walked or worked out every day from diagnosis until after chemo cycle number five. I wanted to work out every day, but I did not have the energy or motivation and could not find it. It is important to stay busy (or at least keep your mind busy) during treatment. You do not want to get lost in your thoughts and spiral. I am both grateful that I worked during treatment and wish that I had had a more flexible schedule. I had a lot going on during treatment. Just before diagnosis, I started a parenting podcast, *Life with Little Ones*, and started interviewing for a new position at within my company. It was overwhelming at times, but I honestly think that it helped me combat chemo brain and kept my mind occupied.

Today I heard the best quote, and it hit differently than any other quote I have ever heard. It is one of those quotes that will live with me forever. "We have two lives, and the second begins when we realize we only have one" (Confucius).

That hit me straight in my heart. I feel like I have had many lives. Your childhood, your adolescence, college years, party years, settle down, get married, and have a baby years. I thought those were lives. When you refer to those times, you say, "Another life ago," and things like that, but during all those year/lives/times, whatever you want to call it, I either thought I was invincible or just did not think of my mortality. I would drink bad thoughts and people away and just keep it moving.

But now I realize that was all one life, that, thank God, I get to bring those lessons with me.

I get this second life, but I get to bring all my memories and lessons. All the survivors that I speak to say you will never be the same. You will never be that person again. At first that made me sad. I sort of kind of *loved* the person I was before. There is always room for improvement, and I was slowly but surely growing up and becoming a better person every day. I was indestructible. I was strong. I was smart and determined. That person and those characteristics got me to where I am now/today. That girl found her dream man, that girl had the son she dreamed up, that girl forced her way into a mammogram at thirty. So, when I realized that she died on the phone with the doctor on September fourth, and my new life started with the very next beat of my heart, it was *heavy* to take on.

Cancer is no joke. In the cancer community, people rate cancers and compare experiences. I can only speak to my experience and my order of treatment. Depending on your type and stage of cancer, your treatment order and treatment plan will be different. Based on my experience, I consider breast cancer and the treatment associated with it dehumanizing.

The first thing to go is your humility, if you have any left, and then your hair. You are examined, and a lot of people must touch your breasts, neck, armpits, and the like. Which is fine. It is in a medical capacity. But then I started to feel detached from my breasts emotionally and mentally. Initially I thought that my right breast had betrayed me and was the reason I was going through all of this. After a little meditation, I realized that my body had not betrayed me. My body had given me warning signs that I did not ignore, and I would need my body to help me get through treatment. I think that is where our mind goes initially: I am sick, so my body betrayed me. That thought process will not help anything, and that mindset will not help you heal more quickly.

I got a short haircut after my first chemo session, on the anniversary of our first date six years prior; I did not want it to be too dramatic when my hair fell out. I wanted the Hallie Berry; everyone at some point has wanted the Hallie Berry. I walked out with the Leslie Jones. To say I was disappointed was an understatement. I tried to take some power back in this situation, and I felt like I had been punched in the gut *again*. Some people do not lose their hair on chemo. So right as the stylist was making the first cut, I was like, *Holy crap, what if my hair does not fall out?* Another spoiler alert: I was not that lucky. It is rare, but it happens to a lucky few, or you can cold cap.

> Cold caps and scalp cooling systems are tightly fitting, strap-on, helmet-type hats filled with a gel coolant that's chilled to between –15 to –40 degrees Fahrenheit. These caps and scalp cooling systems may help some women keep some or quite a bit of their hair during chemotherapy.
>
> Cold caps and scalp cooling systems work by narrowing the blood vessels beneath the skin of the scalp, reducing the amount of chemotherapy medicine that reaches the hair follicles. With less chemotherapy medicine in the follicles, the hair may be less likely to fall out. The cold also decreases the activity of the hair follicles, which slows down cell division and makes the follicles less affected by the chemotherapy medicine.
>
> The cost of using the caps varies depending on the manufacturer, the number of chemotherapy sessions you will be having, and the number of months you will be using the caps. Some users have said the cost of the caps is comparable to the cost of a having a wig made. Check with your insurance carrier to see if the cost of renting the caps is covered." (Uscher 2021)

During each chemotherapy session, you wear the caps or scalp cooling system for twenty to fifty minutes before, during, and after treatment.

I have been informed by breasties that did cold capping that you will still lose hair when you cold cap! You will lose 20 to 30 percent typically. That is normal! It will grow back.

Make absolute certain that your caps fit all the way down on your scalp! Some people don't press down far enough, and the crown of their head does not cool, resulting in a bald spot. Fit them down tightly.

If you use a scalp cooling system during chemotherapy, you must baby your hair during treatment:

- No blow-drying, hot rollers, or straightening irons

- shampoo only every third day with cool water and use a shampoo with no sulfates or parabens

- Keep hair in a loose braid to protect it

- No coloring until three months after chemotherapy is done

- Gentle combing and brushing

After my research and spending so much money on IVF, I decided that cold capping was not for me. Also, there is no guarantee that after going through all of this you would keep all of your hair. So, I bit the bullet and braced myself to lose my hair.

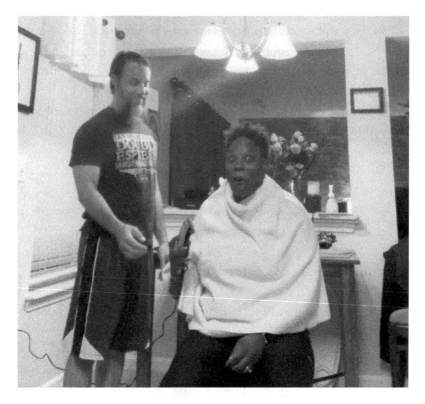

Here we go! Buzz it! Buzz it!

After the second chemo session, my hair started coming out where I had initially had my postnatal hair loss. It was a pandemic, and our kid goes to bed at seven. My hair was falling out, and we were home, so warm up those clippers, baby. My husband shaved my head on Halloween, which just so happens to be my mom's birthday. The irony of the dates is not lost on me. It is just wild. A question that a lot of people want to ask but are too polite or scared to is "Do you miss your hair?"

I do not miss my hair. Not at all. It takes two second to get ready, and I had extensions for over five years, so my wigs are very similar to that. We are in a pandemic, and I do not and cannot go anywhere. I have some turban-like head wraps (from Amazon) that keep my head warm, and I have always loved beanies, so I am all set. I never had to think about my hair being tied to my "beauty" because hair is so whatever. So many people wear wigs, toupees, extensions, or rock a bald head. I was very surprised that losing my hair meant the least to me of all that has happened to date. Hair grows back. I just want to live, but I am glad that my husband was able to do it for me. He surprised me a few days later and shaved his head. My father-in-law also surprised me a couple of days after that and shaved his head. My father-in-law is seventy-five years old and has had the same hair cut for nearly fifty years, so it meant *a lot* that he did that for me. My dad already has a shaved head, so there was nothing to do there. LOL. I am telling you, *get a village*!

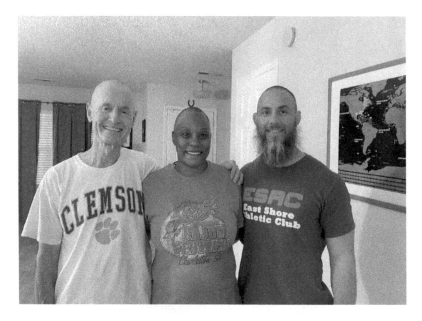

The bald part of my village.

How do the Kardashians or the old ladies at church wear wigs 24-7? Maybe that is why their wigs are often crooked and do not look so great. Wigs are *hot*, and if you are flashing (remember that medically induced menopause) *and* wearing a wig, forget about it. The wig class (a.k.a. lace front tutorial) that I received from my longtime friend Prayer was a legit degree. Learning how to lay edges, dying the lace, tinting the part, how to glue down a wig, making sure I know when I can and should wear synthetic versus real hair. I am just glad that I needed my wigs in the winter. I honestly did not wear wigs as often as I thought I would. In the pandemic and being immunocompromised, I could not leave the house as much as would have wished and

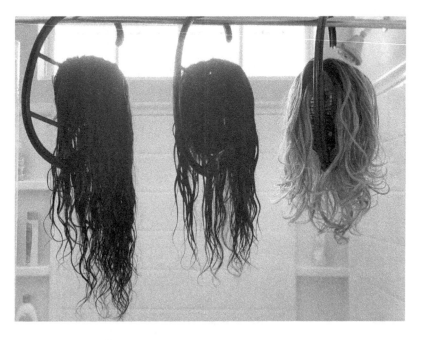

A few of my wigs—a girl needs options

While undergoing chemo, you are pumped full of poison. Let me pause here. Please do not misunderstand; I am grateful for the poison. I am grateful that my cancer was caught early. I am grateful that I was raised to ask questions and ask again if I did not understand a run-around answer that was given to me. I am grateful to have this second life. I am grateful for everything from my first life. But I do not wish cancer on my worst enemy.

The poison does unmentionable things to your body. To list a few:

- Nausea

- Mouth Sores

- Vomiting

- Diarrhea

- Hair loss (everywhere)

- Loss of appetite

- Fatigue

- Fever

- Pain

- Constipation

- Easy bruising

- Bleeding

I did not lose my eyebrows, eyelashes, or arm hair until after I finished chemo. The arm hair part is always so weird to me; it never went anywhere. It held on and stuck in there. All the other hair on my body took a hike right after the second round of chemo.

My side effects included: hair loss, nose bleeds, neuropathy, fatigue, loss of appetite, diarrhea, bruising, severe acid reflux, and pretty bad snoring. I never threw up once. My nose bled so badly all day every day that Trey had to buy me those cotton nosebleed plugs like I was a professional football player. We had to stain treat and wash our sheets every morning.

I got sad for about two days a week. I am on antianxiety meds but not depression meds. Never wanted that. I do not know if I needed them but will not ask. This week I think I was sad I could not get treatment sooner and that I have no quantifiable evidence that I am getting better. I have very minimal side effects from the chemo, thank God, but then I go down a rabbit hole of am I being healed? Are they giving me the right medicine?

I oddly *love* chemo day. This is the only day in a three-week period that I feel that I am actively killing the cancer.

11.19.20

> I am still sad. And now I am embarrassed I just cried in the chemo room. Eh, it is whatever. Trying not to be a downer. I am in the waiting room waiting on blood results and the doc. Yup, cleared for cycle 3. Love you. I'm just scared.

The hurry up and wait took a toll on me during chemo. I hit a small wall before chemo number four. At halfway through chemo, my emotions were getting the best of me.

12.9.20

I had a hard last two nights. I do not know what happens to me at night. I guess the weight of it all finally hits me when I sit down for the day. How much further I have to go. How my looks have already changed. I have never cried so hard. I think Trey was almost scared. Like, dude, I am bald and gaining and losing weight in weird places, and I am going to have scars everywhere, and I am so far from being done. It is like, hurry up and wait. And what if it is spreading now or whatever. Like I am just so sad and scared. And it sucks to just keep on keeping on like nothing is happening. The world keeps spinning. It all keeps coming, and I am supposed to do it all? IDK.

There are so many questions, and I am also straddling a line of wanting to be informed and being my own health-care advocate and being too demanding. Everyone is on my team. I have hand-selected my doctors and my team, and they have done everything—and more than—I have asked. I do not know; I am just a little lost. I want to be done with chemo. I want mental clarity and to have the mental strength to be there for someone else. Right now, I am just nearly crippled with fear to even post about my own cancer because I do not want it to get worse, and I have to post an update. That is *so* stupid, but those are my thoughts. These are the ramblings of someone who has not slept in twenty-four hours due to the middle-of-the-night diarrhea attacks.

I am tired of being strong, but I will not and cannot stop.

The rest of chemo went well after I learned my limits and what I needed to do when. Everyone is different, and your treatment will be different. The first round of chemo will be terrible, but when you learn your own limitations and needs, it will fly by. You will not remember everything that you think you will. There is also chemo brain, so all through treatment, and not just chemo, take notes, journal, and ask questions.

At the end of chemo, you have an MRI to look at your lesion (a.k.a. tumor) to see if it responded to the chemo and so your doctor can make some decisions before surgery. My MRI looked great. I then had my last chemo cycle, and I graduated chemo. The facility had an outside courtyard that was right off of the chemo suite, so my family was able to come to watch me ring the bell. That was one of the best days of my life. I did not cry, though. It did not feel real. I cry when I see others ring the bell, and I thought I would cry, but I did not. I also falsely had a sense of completion; I think the MRI results contributed to that too.

About a week later, I had one of the worst days of my life. A lot of highs and lows. I went to the restroom, and I thought it was going to be diarrhea. I was bleeding out of my rectum. It was so painful that I was crying, and I felt like I was going to throw up at the same time. I honestly had my phone in my hand and could not figure out whether to call my husband in the other room or call 911. My brain completely shut down. I was in the restroom for over an hour. That was the culmination and accumulation of chemo for me.

Thank God this happened after I finished treatment. I never understood how people could just *not* go to treatment or stop before completing their treatment plan. My anxiety would eat me alive; I would be in "trouble" with my oncologist and mom! But I did not have that experience, during all of treatment, with my side effects, and then it dawned on me that many people do have that experience with treatment, and my mind was blown.

But that is why ringing the bell is a little problematic. It mentally gives you a false sense of completion. It was my choice to ring the bell in January, and I do not regret it. I just wish I had realized that there were over four months of concentrated chemo in my system, and I wish I had taken it a little easier off the bat. I have heard discussions of removing bells from chemo and radiation, but a lot of people need that validation. *I did!* But it has become problematic lately. Imagine if you are metastatic or have an incurable cancer and while you are sitting there receiving treatment you keep seeing people ring their bells. That would make me really sad, and I did not think about that until after the fact. I do not have type A questions for chemo because you have to attend chemo teach (a.k.a. chemo school), and they give you a book/binder with everything you will need. Make sure to get your own binder, around three inches. You will want to keep everything anyone gives you and keep it organized.

I will be continuing on with immunotherapy until September. Immunotherapy is nothing like chemo. I only get one drug, Herceptin, and it does not make me sick. I do not have any side effects to mention, and my hair can grow back too!

Type A Tips for Chemo

- Take a bag for things you will need for a full day.

    - I took a roller suitcase with my laptop, iPad, phone, all charging cords, cordless headphones, snacks, and ice water.

- Try to move at least once a day, even if it is a short walk.

- Nap, nap, nap!

- Stay hydrated.

- If you are able to, go in for fluids on chemo off-weeks.

- Eat what you can when you can, but you will want to try to eat brain-boosting foods.

    - The side effects from chemo may prevent you from eating like you used to, but do what you can.

    - Use plastic cutlery to avoid emphasizing the metallic taste of food.

- If you need to cry, *cry*!

- If you need to scream, *scream*!

- If you are able, find an oncological therapist.

- If you have bad diarrhea, make pad cycles if you need relief. If you have not had a baby, no worries—Google it.

- Consider cold capping to conserve your hair. I did not do that, but it is a personal choice.

- Ice your fingers and toes—it cuts down on neuropathy.

    · I did not do it, and I am going on two months of pain in my fingers.

    · You can also suck on ice or a popsicle to help with this.

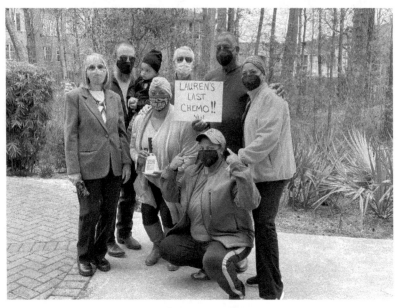

Chemo Graduation

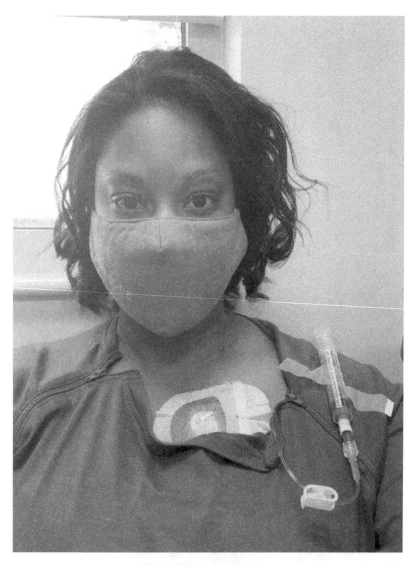

First Day of Chemo

CHAPTER 8:

Surgery

The weeks following chemo were filled with more highs and lows. The MRI looked great, but I would not know if I was NED (no evidence of disease, a.k.a. cancer-free) until the pathology results from surgery, and that was six weeks away. That was a little difficult. I would have a stretch of good days and then have a complete meltdown. I did not and do not want to die from this. I am young, too young. It made me skittish. I started to hate this timid and scared person I had become. I had to decide on what surgery I was going to have, as well as what kind of reconstruction to have. A lot of women are not told that they can choose to go flat after a single or double mastectomy. Your treatment is your choice from beginning to end. You do not have to have reconstruction if you do not want to. I recommend listening to your doctor's suggestions, but I have a saying: The doctor knows cancer better than you do, but you know *you* better than anyone.

Your treatment plan should be a conversation, not your doctor talking at you.

I decided to have a bilateral mastectomy instead of a single mastectomy.

First, my doctor said that the chance of getting cancer in my remaining breast was 7 to 9 percent, and that seemed like too much for me. Also, the surgeon said that my natural breasts were so large that it would be harder—not impossible, but a lot harder than normal—to get symmetrical results with a reduction and lift on the remaining breast. Second, my son had eczema as an infant, and as one does, we tried a lot of things to try to solve it. Accordingly, he had to go on formula at four months old. A fed baby is best, so in my opinion I did not need to keep my left breast to feed future children. My number one priority was to be around for them.

In the six-week period between finishing chemo and my bilateral mastectomy, I just immersed myself in work, the podcast, and getting my body and home ready for surgery. We made and froze meals. We signed up for meal delivery services, and we got a bidet! Those things may not seem like they are related, but they are. I usually do most of the cooking, while Trey does all of the grilling, but after surgery, when we would be taking care of me and our two-year-old son, whom I could not pick up for six to eight weeks, we needed dinner time to be as seamless as possible. I didn't know what range of motion or abilities I would have after surgery, and to keep the magic alive in our marriage, we don't need to know how the sausage is made. He didn't look below the equator when I gave birth to our son, and I did not want Trey to literally have to wipe my butt, so we got a bidet! Win, win, win!

2.25.21

Today is Thursday, and I am five days away from my double mastectomy, and I am scared shitless, to be honest. I want to live, and I want to be here for Chip and our popsicle babies and possible other future children.

The day before surgery, I had to go to the hospital to get my lymph nodes mapped for removal as well as get a shot of dye into my areola for surgery prep. That was wild and uncomfortable, to say the least. Before all this cancer mess, I had only had Lasik, some dental surgery, and my port surgery. Now I am staring down the barrel of full anesthesia.

I baked cookies for the nurses at the hospital and wrote them a note that I laminated; I also laminated a photo of Chip to the back of the letter. I introduced myself and made myself seem more human versus just a patient. I told them about my diagnosis and my family and to resuscitate me by any means necessary.

3.2.21

A letter to my nurses.

My name is Lauren. I know that I may be out of it, but I think there may be information that you may need from me.

Thank you in advance for being here for me in lieu of my family and being my nurse(s).

It really sucks due to COVID-19 that my husband could not be here and stay; but it is what it is, and we are where we are.

If you need to reach him:

His name is Trey, and his phone number is xxx-xxx-xxxx.

I have a two-year-old son named Chip, and his birthday was two days ago!

Resuscitate please. I want to live no matter what.

I am a Libra; my favorite food is sushi and/or anything Italian.

I was diagnosed with stage 2 HER2-positive breast cancer last year, when I was thirty-four. That kind of messed up my life plans.

I have a sequin turban in my bag. I would like to wear that for at least a little bit, please.

If I get cold, I have a hot pink CC beanie. I am too bald not to have anything on my head. LOL.

I know y'all know what you are doing, but this is a major surgery. I have only had one other, for my port, so I am a little scared.

I hope I am not out of it too much.

I have made cookies for each shift, as a thank you in advance, and they are labeled!

xxo Lauren

The morning of my surgery, I was very scared. I was trying to be strong for Trey, my family, and everyone texting. I was making jokes in pre-op and per usual talking my head off. I was just trying to distract myself.

I will never forget the way that Trey looked at me when he had to leave. I know that he loves me and our son. In all that we have been through in our life together and with cancer, he has never looked at me like this. It was a look of pity, empathy, and fear. I could see in his eyes that he saw my fear, even though my jokes, and I could see that he did not want me to die. I had to catch my breath, and my heart skipped a beat. I was just really trying not to cry, and that moment lasted for a long time and happened in slow motion. For some reason I thought it would be funny to tell him I would see him later in Spanish: "Hasta luego, mi amor; te amo," and I do not remember anything else until waking up in my hospital room ten hours later.

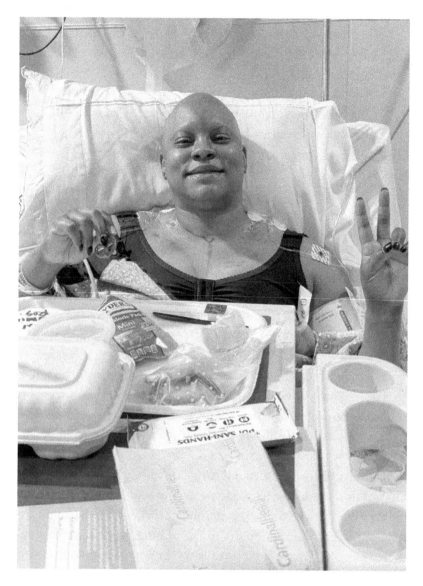

First photo post double mastectomy.

This is not a boob job. A bilateral mastectomy is not a boob job; it is more like an amputation. I know that a lot of people do not know what to say when you talk about having to have a body part removed, but it is not a boob job, and it certainly is not free. I have no feeling across my chest, my right armpit, and in parts of my back. It is unknown if the feeling will return. There is so much unknown. I think that is why I am so skeptical about this whole process. There are so many things that the doctors are sure about, and there is still a lot they do not know.

My surgery went well. My surgeons worked in tandem. My oncological surgeon started on the right, and the plastic surgeon went to the right breast once she was finished. The surgery was supposed to take about four hours, but it took nearly eight hours. There was a snafu with one of my expanders. It was punctured, and they had to find another. Also, I ended up having nine out of twenty-three lymph nodes removed. But all was well, and I woke up starving and looking for my husband.

The recovery from the bilateral mastectomy was not nearly as hard as I thought it would be. When I was first diagnosed, Emily came over and talked me through her journey and told me that chemo would be the hardest thing I had to do and all subsequent treatments would be easier than the last. And she was right. Chemo and the side effects were hard. Surgery was not that bad; it is just awkward to not to use your arms and to sleep in a position like you are in a body cast. A lot of people sleep in recliners, but I slept in our bed. I bought wedge pillows and a reading pillow. The worst two things post-surgery were my throat hurting from the tube and the neuropathy, weakness, numbness, and pain, usually in the hands and feet. It can also affect other areas of your body. That came in hot after surgery. There are side effects that show up months after chemo; the main two are neuropathy and chemo brain. My chemo brain was exacerbated by the anesthesia, and it was pretty bad for about a week or two.

I will say that the best part, or, I guess, the most pleasant surprise, was the ON-Q pump that I woke up with. "Your ON-Q pump will continuously deliver a local anesthetic medication to block the pain in the area of your procedure. As the medication is delivered, the pump ball will gradually become smaller. Because the pump delivers the medication very slowly, it's not uncommon for it to take up to 24 hours before you'll notice a change in the size and look of the pump" (myon-q.com 2018). When I got home from the hospital, I already had not slept for thirty-six hours; anesthesia will mess you up like that. The pain killers they were giving me did not put me to sleep. So, I was a zombie, and that will make you emotional as is. Though I had not slept, I barely had any pain. I attribute that to nerve blockers and the ON-Q system.

At my three-day checkup, the ON-Q Pump was removed, and they took my bandages off. I saw my "new" breasts, or what was left of them. I went from a 36 E to a B cup at best; they filled my expanders with air after surgery. That was the most jarring. I wish someone had told me do not worry what they looked like right then. "They will resemble breasts in two weeks; do not worry." No one told me that. It is not anyone's fault. I just reacted. It was a lot.

I had to have lymph nodes removed too, so there is an area between my breast and armpit that is concave. It is a drastic change, and it made me sad. I felt incomplete and mutilated at the same time. I felt hacked, dehumanized. In addition to feeling terrible from no sleep, I did not have more than two-hour sleep stints for five days; I did not recognize this person in the mirror. I went from having my annual mammogram to quiet the anxious voices in my head to being positive for cancer to having my eggs harvested to going through the ringer with chemo. Losing my hair, and now losing my breasts.

My hair, breasts, and fertility did not and do not define me or a woman, but they were part of my identity, right? When you have a mastectomy, you are asked if you want to spare your nipples, and there should be a discussion about whether you are able to. I was able but decided not to. I was told that they would not have sensation and may not even work. The 3D nipple tattoo industry has grown by leaps and bounds in the last few years. That will be my last stop after I am finished with treatment!

Cancer is the great equalizer. In the beginning everyone looks like their old self. But as treatment continues, you go through a transformation. Mentally, emotionally, and physically. I am speaking from my own experience, but I know I lost myself. Again, I did not recognize the woman in the mirror. You either lose or gain weight; I did both. I lost twenty pounds after my diagnosis and first chemo treatment. Then I gained forty pounds from steroids, fluids, and everything else they were pumping me full of. And then you lose your hair. When it all hits you, you are staring at a bald stranger with a round face and a pot belly in the mirror. I get winded from crying and going up the stairs. *Who am I? Who is this?*

In my darkest days after surgery, I realized that I was grieving again. I had kept myself so busy leading up to surgery to I had not allowed myself time to grieve. At my lowest I did not just pray; I spoke openly and audibly to God. I asked, for the first time, *why?* Why me? What can I do for you? How are you using me as a vehicle? What message do you want me to convey? Why did you have to take me down to the studs to have me deliver this message?

I cried myself to sleep that night waiting for an answer. The next day I realized that my mind and body were going to heal at about the same pace. Every day I get stronger mentally and physically; please believe me when I say, it gets better!

Two weeks out from surgery, and these have been a hard two weeks. I did not foresee them being so hard.

3.19.21

I had my first fill of my expanders today. Sometimes during a mastectomy, they will go straight to implants. I was not that lucky; also, I believe my doctor did that due to my need for radiation. When they fill your expander for the first time, they must take the air out of the expander that they put in at the time of surgery; they replace it with saline. When my doctor deflated the expanders, it looked like deflated soufflés. It was wild.

Then he filled them. My chest is numb, so it did not hurt. He had also taken out the stitches. I have never had surgery, so this is all new to me.

On my first fill, I got 450 ccs; he says that does not translate to cup size. Dr Google says that translates to a C cup. For my peace of mind, I will go with Dr. Google today.

A week later I went in for a second fill; they took out one of my surgical drains then too. I did not mind my drains. It is something else to do, and you must track how much drainage you are putting out, and they are a little itchy, but other than that, it just is what it is.

4.6.21

Today I am five weeks from surgery, and I feel like a new woman. Both of my drains have been taken out, and I am off of the antibiotics and the nerve blockers, so my permanent haze of nausea is gone! I feel like I have done a one-eighty. Every day it gets better. Please remember that. It is ok to have bad days, but they will not last.

Please note that drains are a necessary evil. They are itchy and sometimes hurt, and they make it impossible to sleep in a normal position, but they were fine. If you get them taken out too early, it can have serious consequences. The drains help the excess fluid drain away so that you can heal faster and more efficiently. If you get your drains taken out too soon, you can develop an abscess or a seroma.

Incision and drainage are a minor surgical procedure for removing fluid buildup from under the skin or infected sinuses. It is commonly performed to treat several types of hematomas, seromas, and other soft tissue infections that lead to fluid accumulation. This procedure is also referred to as IND or I&D.

Incision and drainage are performed to release the pressure caused by the production of excess fluid, one of the body's immune response to infection. I&D is often con-current with antibiotics therapy, especially if the risk of developing bacterial infection following the procedure is high. (DocDoc n.d.)

If you were to develop a bacterial infection, then you may have to get your expander emptied or even removed while you heal. Same if you have already had your exchange surgery and you are having this is-sue with an implant; you may have to get your implant removed and the whole process started over again after you have healed from the infection.

Please think twice and ask your doctor a lot of questions when it comes to your drains; it is very important.

Type A Questions to Ask Your Surgeon

- How long will it take me to recover?

- Confirm your procedure:

    · Lumpectomy

    · Single mastectomy

    · Double mastectomy

- What are the permanent side effects?

- Am I able to keep my nipples?

  - Is there an increased chance of recurrence if I do keep them?

- What are the side effects?

- Is it possible to have an ON-Q pump?

- Will I have drains?

  - How many?

  - For how long?

- Discuss scar and incision options.

  - Across the breast or anchor style?

- Where will I lose feeling?

  - Do you know if the feeling will return?

- Will I need to stay in the hospital?

  - How long?

Type A Tips for Surgery

- Before surgery, practice standing up without using your hands and arms.

- Get meals ready and put in the freezer to save time and effort later.

- Reach out to your village and see what kind of time and services people have to offer.

- Continue to exercise, within your limits, until surgery.

- Get mastectomy pillows for your car rides; usually these are donated to the hospital and provided at no charge to you.

- You will not be able to drive for a bit; for double mastectomy patients, arrange transportation for follow-up appointments.

- Make sure to get a lanyard or a belt for your drains so they have somewhere to rest and a way to be secured.

- Shower seats are helpful, but I stayed with the birdbaths. I stayed away from the shower and baths.

- They will give you a surgical bra, but I bought additional front-close bras for cleanliness and comfort.

- Stay on top of your meds per your doctor's instructions. By the time you feel pain, it'll take a bit to reside.

- Do not ice your chest. You need increased circulation to heal best, and ice slows down circulation.

CHAPTER 9:

Radiation

Why do I need radiation if I have already had a complete response to chemo and a double mastectomy?

Radio therapy uses high doses of radiation to kill cancer cells, and when used after surgery and chemotherapy, as in my case, it is used to kill any remaining microscopic cancer cells. Also, since my cancer had spread to my lymph nodes, I required radiation to reduce the risk that cancer could recur there.

In studies it has shown to reduce recurrence and increase survival rates, and I feel comfortable with what the doctor and I discussed. But it was not easy, and I did not get there right off the bat.

Radiation was one of the largest hills I had to climb. I did not want to do this. I was not having a great day, and we went to see the radiologist, and she broke down the most common and some less common side effects of radiation:

- Fatigue

- Burns

- Hair loss

- Skin changes

- Swelling (edema)

- Tenderness

- Shortness of breath

The radiologist also told me that my ribs would receive a small amount of treatment, so for the rest of my life, my ribs would be a little more fragile on the right side versus the left. There was less than a 5 percent chance, but I could also develop a different kind of cancer from the radiation itself. That day was not the day. I declared that I would not be getting radiation, and I called my oncological surgeon, my oncologist, and Ebony.

I went home, I rested, and I contemplated. No one could make me do radiation, and no one in my village had gone through it, so they did not really know what to say. I got on social media to mentally unplug, and I came across a post from a metastatic baddie that I follow. And her positivity on that post, and her positivity in general, stopped me in my tracks. I needed to check myself and my privilege, and that is exactly what I did. I am a black woman in America, and we are one of the least regarded groups of people in the country. I have a team and village of people fighting for me. They are not fighting the same fight as I, but we are on the same side, and they want me to be successful. I have insurance that is going to pay for me to receive this treatment. I need to take all the treatment I can when it is instructed so that I can nip this whole yearlong detour in the bud. Who am I to refuse any treatment?

Yes, I am tired. Yes, I feel slightly hacked up and mutilated, but this was always part of the journey. I had been told since day one with Dr. D that I would be receiving radiation. All the treatment had side effects, some terrible, some tolerable, and this was one of the last treatments.

So here we go. Twenty-five sessions of external radiation to my chest wall and axillary lymph nodes to finish this. With my drains finally out, I could get mapped for radiation.

I was instructed to undress fully on the top and that the nurse would come back in the room. The table was confusing, and in my usual fashion, I lay on the table incorrectly. I had my feet on the handlebars. I thought the nurse was going to pee her pants when she saw me, and I looked like I was about to work out and do sit-ups or work out on a rowing machine. There was a beanbag-like material that they put under me. They asked me to put my arm up, and then they sucked the air out of the "beanbag" to make the mold (a.k.a. cradle) that I would lie in every time I came in. I also received a CT of my chest wall and armpit. They lined up the laser and drew markings on me where I would be receiving the treatment with a tattoo marker and covered that with see-through waterproof bandages. Back to not scrubbing or being able to submerge yourself in water again for another six weeks, back to the birdbaths and quick showers.

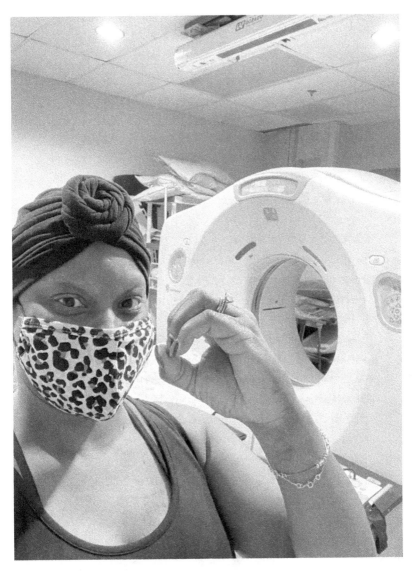

Mapping prep for radiation.

4.20.21

I already have been down a shame spiral of feeling stupid after actually thinking of not doing radiation. Today was a breeze. The first one is always the hardest. But I need to stop getting so wrapped up and listen to my predecessors. Each treatment is less invasive than the last. Every day gets better and easier.

One down; twenty-four to go. I had my second Moderna shot yesterday and first radio therapy session today, and I feel invincible. I can see the finish line. I feel like if I had blown off radiation, I would have been taking a cab to the finish line. That is not to say that if you were not prescribed radiation, this has anything to do with you. It is just this was prescribed and suggested for me, and it is my part of my job to complete this therapy. I have a total of six lotions-it is a lot of lotion-and cannot wait to check this off the list too. I have so much support I am nearly emotional. Thank you, everyone who is here for and with me. All I see is the women in my family past and present standing as pillars for me in the instances where I feel weak. This is not to say that if you are not in my family, I do not see you. This is to say that if you are in my healing village, I consider you family.

What do I know? I do not know anything about this. All the research I did before this, I am currently feeling is pointless. Everyone's experience is different, and I hate that. I need consistency, and I would like to get this part of treatment under control as much as I have the other parts of treatment. It is day two, and I did lotion up, but they ask me to do it twice a day, and I did it once. I am just a little lost, and the people are nice, but I am in my feelings. I am nervous, and I need a little coddling. I will never let them know that. I have only cried once since leaving there after easily seven appointments.

I am just feeling pitiful today, and I will be asleep soon enough. I am just ready for this to be over, but there are around 190 days left

Insert eye roll here.

5.10.12

We have just returned from our first family vacation since January 2020. We went up to a local beach for a family member's outdoor wedding. It was a lot of fun, and I loved seeing everyone, but I am beat. I thought it was from the drinking and celebrations, but I now know that it is from the radiation. I thought I would do better-not that it is a competition, but I did so well with all the other treatments there, was no way a little radiation was going to take me down. I changed my deodorant very early on to one without aluminum. I have been using all the creams the doctor and people who have had radiation before me advised me to use. Some people told me they didn't get tired at all. The fatigue comes and goes; it feels very similar to chemo fatigue, but it's a solo symptom. It does not come with the nose bleeds and stomach stuff.

On Mondays they measure me. Measure to make sure the beams are hitting the correct and same spots. On Tuesdays they x-ray me. Making sure everything looks good inside. On Wednesdays I see the doctor, and she checks my skin. She tells me I am doing well so far. Today was session fifteen of twenty-five. I am 60 percent done and very excited. I do feel like I am about to hit a wall.

I feel guilty when I get to this point. I want to be positive and have gratitude so that I can make this process as easy on the body and mind as possible, but that is what toxic positivity is. You can't fake feeling good or positive during something like this. I felt like this after the fourth chemo session, four days after surgery, and now just over halfway through radiation. Cancer is hard. I do not have the luxury of being selfish at this time. My husband is my caretaker, and he is fantastic, but I feel bad when I just need to sleep. Chip doesn't understand that Mommy can't just play at the drop of a dime. Today after radiation I passed out for three hours. I needed it, but I have mom-guilt, wife-guilt, and just guilt.

5/13/21

I spoke too soon. The skin in my armpit is burned black, and the veins in my right breast are purple and very apparent. It doesn't hurt because I still don't have feeling in my breasts and part of my back. I was instructed by the doctor to increase the frequency of how many times I apply lotion, and we just need to get past these last six sessions. I hopped out of the car today headed to treatment, and instantly I thought there was a fifteen-year-old with poor hygiene sneaking up behind me; it was just me and my armpits stinking due to the natural deodorant that I have been forced to switch to.

Note to self: you can use the regular deodorant in the armpit that is not receiving radiation.

I finished radiation on a Monday. My doctor said I tolerated radio therapy well, I was skeptical; my armpit, and the skin under my breast and part of my back, are all the way black. Not just darker, like, oh, you had fun on vacation and forgot sunscreen—*black* like Mom burnt dinner, and we can't even air out the house fast enough, so we are going to Outback. Some people get blisters and all the symptoms of an intense sunburn; so, I guess I *did* handle it well.

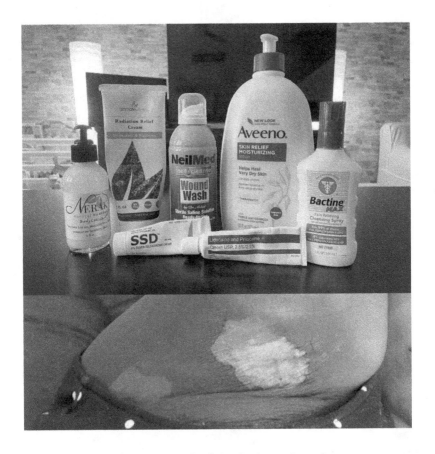

Radiation burn relief products and my burn.

We went out to eat on Saturday and Monday. Eh, I am cancer-free; what are you going to do? We have gotten a lot better about celebrating the little things and each milestone. I think that is best. If you are diagnosed in September and you do not celebrate anything for a year (or after you are finished with treatment), that is a long haul of treatment and a lot of accomplishments gone by the wayside.

Do what you would like, of course, but I am going to celebrate—a lot.

Type A Guide to Questions to Ask your Radiologist

- How many sessions will I require?

- How will you map/mark me?

- Are the marks permanent?

- What type of radio therapy will I receive—internal or external?

- What are the side effects?

- Where will I be receiving my radio therapy?

- How many days a week do you do treatment, five or seven?

- Can I receive radiation more than once in my lifetime?

Type A Tips for Radiation

- Keep your treated area out of direct sunlight.

- Make sure the lotion or aloe you are using for treatment does not contain alcohol.

- Get more than one type of lotion.

- Ask people with similar skin types and colors what they used.

- Keep track of how many sessions you will have.

- Figure out what schedule for treatment works for you.

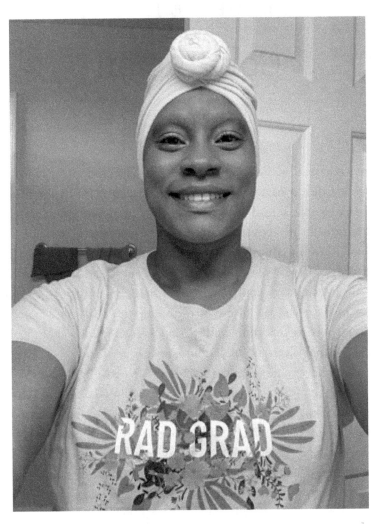

Radiation Graduation Day!

CHAPTER 10:

Conclusion

I do not have all the answers. What I have is a road map / blueprint of what I did to navigate my cancer, treatment plan, the grant and insurance systems. I still have questions and need some guidance with posttreatment life specific to nutrition, mental health, and the day-to-day. Most specifically, how do I navigate daily life with all the knowledge I have about things that cause cancer?

We live in a very confusing world where companies and the government allow the sale of products and services that cause cancer. I am not referring to alcohol and cigarettes. I am talking about make-up, acrylic nails, certain foods, and hair care products.

I have never really thought I was *great* at anything. If you ask my best friend, my friends, or my family, they will disagree, but I always feel like I come up short. I do not say this for you to feel bad for me, but I always feel like I am lacking. So, when there is something, I do well, I kind of overdo it. I do not usually bow out on a high note. That is something I should tackle in the rest of my thirties.

But I talk a lot, and I think maybe that is what I do well (if you can talk a lot well). Maybe this is so I can help people detect their cancer early or ignite a flame inside someone that will end up curing cancer, after they realize how debilitating this disease is. I think people expect older people or people who smoke to get cancer. And when this happens to those groups of people, it is not as jarring and doesn't feel as "unfair" as when a younger person who doesn't do those things gets cancer.

Bad things are not normal, and we should destigmatize trauma and pain. If someone makes it to the age of one hundred, we should still be fazed and bothered if they get cancer. The statistics for cancer are disconcerting, and we need to change this *now*. It is wild to me that cancer has become so commonplace. Bad things have become daily occurrences that do not shake us as much as they once did. Life-consuming grief is not normal. Why should I be expected to act as if this huge life-changing moment has not consumed and derailed thirteen months of my short life?

People in positions of power and companies that want our money should be protecting us, not using us up until we do not have any money left, experience dire side effects, or die from their products and move onto the next.

We as survivors are expected to just go back to life as if nothing happened. As if we have not had an additional full-time job for the last year. All emotions, feelings, and fears are to be pushed down and ignored. And if not, you are the cancer girl, and that is worse than the accountant that has to lie about their job at parties.

As a survivor I feel like I am more of an oversharer than I was before, and I have got to watch that. Some people do not want to hear about *all* of your side effects (diarrhea) when they ask, "How you're doing?"

To get by you will need to laugh and/or cry daily, and that is ok. Feelings will surface from time to time that you did not know you were still feeling or holding on to, and that is ok too! I still cry, and I feel better for it afterward. I used to be embarrassed to cry like this, but I have flipped my perspective.

Now I am just grateful to feel.

This is not going to be a neat ending because cancer does not usually have a nice, neat ending. It is ongoing and will require monitoring for the rest of my life. My future comes with a lot of scans, monitoring, a little Xanax, some red wine, and an air of uncertainty.

Keep up with me on @typeaguidetocancer on Instagram, the podcast *Life with Little Ones* and www.typeaguidetocancer.com

Last word

Stay strong

FU, cancer

Love,

Lauren

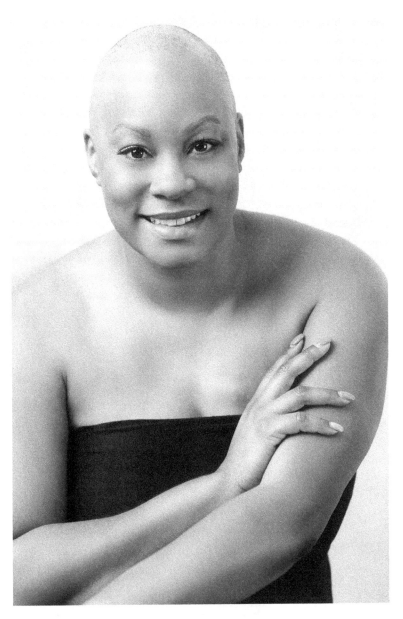

"With Gratitude...Lauren T."

Glossary

AYA cancer—adolescent and young adult (AYA) cancer is any cancer that impacts a person aged fifteen to thirty-nine at the time of diagnosis.

breast cancer—breast cancer is cancer that forms in the cells of the breasts. After skin cancer, breast cancer is the most common cancer diagnosed in women in the United States. Breast cancer can occur in both men and women, but it's far more common in women.

benign—not cancerous (a.k.a. not malignant).

bilateral mastectomy—the surgical removal of both breasts to treat or prevent breast cancer. There are several reasons why a patient might need or choose to undergo this procedure.

biopsy—an examination of tissue removed from a living body to discover the presence, cause, or extent of a disease.

BRCA gene—What Is BRCA? The name "BRCA" is an abbreviation for "BReast CAncer gene." BRCA1 and BRCA2 are two different genes that have been found to impact a person's chances of developing breast cancer.

cancer—a disease caused by an uncontrolled division of abnormal cells in a part of the body.

cancer staging—staging is the process of finding out how much cancer is in a person's body and where it's located. It's how the doctor determines the stage of a person's cancer. https://www.cancer.org/treatment/understanding-your-diagnosis/staging.html.

chemotherapy—the treatment of disease by the use of chemical substances, especially the treatment of cancer by cytotoxic and other drugs.

chemo port—a small, implantable reservoir with a thin silicone tube that attaches to a vein. The main advantage of this vein-access device is that chemotherapy medications can be delivered directly into the port rather than a vein, eliminating the need for needle sticks. https://moffitt.org/treatments/chemotherapy/what-is-a-chemo-port/.

CT Scan—an X-ray image made using a form of tomography in which a computer controls the motion of the X-ray source and detectors, processes the data, and produces the image.

diagnosis—the identification of the nature of an illness or other problem by examination of the symptoms.

echocardiogram (echo)—a graphic outline of the heart's movement. During an echo test, ultrasound (high-frequency sound waves) from a handheld wand placed on your chest provides pictures of the heart's valves and chambers and helps the sonographer evaluate the pumping action of the heart.

fertility specialist—diagnoses and treats problems related to infertility. If you have been trying to get pregnant for a year (or six months if you are over thirty-five) and natural conception is not working, a fertility specialist can diagnose and treat your problems.

genetic testing—the sequencing of human DNA in order to discover genetic differences, anomalies, or mutations that may prove pathological.

GP—general physician

immunotherapy—the prevention or treatment of disease with substances that stimulate the immune response.

invasive ductal carcinoma (IDC)—the most common type of breast cancer. About 80 percent of all breast cancers are invasive ductal carcinomas.

IVF—in vitro fertilization

lymph nodes—small lumps of tissue that contain white blood cells that fight infection.

mammography—specialized medical imaging that uses a low-dose X-ray system to see inside the breasts. A mammography exam is called a mammogram.

Malignant—(of a tumor) tending to invade normal tissue or to recur after removal; cancerous.

MRI—magnetic resonance imaging; a form of medical imaging that measures the response of the atomic nuclei of body tissues to high-frequency radio waves when placed in a strong magnetic field and that produces images of the internal organs.

oncology—the study of cancer

PET scan—an image made using positron emission tomography, especially one of the brain

PCP—primary care provider

seroma—buildup of fluid under the surface of the skin at the surgical site, weeks after the surgery itself. It is considered one of the body's responses to tissue removal.

surgical drain—a thin, flexible rubber tube into the area of your body where the fluid is likely to collect. The rubber tube carries the fluid out of your body into a collection bulb that you empty.

treatment plan—layout of the expected path of treatment. It is a document that is created by the cancer care team and given to the patient and others that may need to know the planned course of care.

tumor—a swelling of a part of the body, generally without inflammation, caused by an abnormal growth of tissue, whether benign or malignant

survivor—a person who continues to function or prosper in spite of opposition, hardship, or setbacks.

warrior—a person who shows or has shown great vigor, courage, or aggressiveness

Bibliography

Cancer Disparities in the Black Community. 2020. Accessed April 12, 2021. https://www.cancer.org/about-us/what-we-do/health-equity/cancer-disparities-in-the-black-community.html.

DocDoc. n.d. Accessed March 29, 2021. https://www.docdoc.com/medical-information/procedures/incision-and-drainage-of-hematoma-seroma-or-fluid-collection.

Healthline.com. 2018. What is a PET Scan? August 27. Accessed February 17, 2021. https://www.healthline.com/health/pet-scan.

Klein, Amy. 2020. IVF Treatment Costs Guide. April 18. Accessed March 21, 2021. https://www.nytimes.com/article/ivf-treatment-costs-guide.html.

Mayo Clinic Staff. 2019. Tests-Procedures. Accessed March 18, 2021. https://www.mayoclinic.org/tests-procedures/in-vitro-fertilization/about/pac-20384716.

myon-q.com. 2018. Accessed May 21, 2021. https://myon-q.com/on-q-pump/.

National Breast Cancer Foundation. 2020. What is BRCA. April 15. Accessed March 19, 2021. https://www.nationalbreastcancer.org/what-is-brca#:~:text=What%20Is%20BRCA%3F,chances%20of%20developing%20breast%20cancer.

National Cancer Institute. 2020. AYA . September 24. Accessed February 10, 2021. https://www.cancer.gov/types/aya.

Stupid Cancer. 2021. Instagram Post. April 1.

uclahealth.org/ayacancer. 2021. Accessed March 1, 2021. https://www.uclahealth.org/ayacancer/.

Uscher, Jen. 2021. Cold Caps and Scalp Cooling Systems. May 14. Accessed May 17, 2021. https://www.breastcancer.org/treatment/side_effects/hair-loss/cold-caps-scalp-cooling.

What Are My Options. 2020. Accessed April 2, 2021. https://resolve.org/what-are-my-options/insurance-coverage/infertility-coverage-state/#:~:text=As%20of%20August%202020%2C%2019,(medically%2Dinduced)%20infertility.

who.int. 2020. COVID-19. Accessed March 3, 2021. https://www.who.int/emergencies/diseases/novel-coronavirus-2019/question-and-answers-hub/q-a-detail/coronavirus-disease-covid-19.

Wikipedia. 2020. Accessed March 5, 2021. https://en.wikipedia.org/wiki/COVID-19.

Doctor's Notes

Doctor's Notes